EXPECTING EXCELLENCE IN PARENTING

A Comprehensive Guide to Nurturing Exceptional Child and Creating Lasting Bonds

PATRICIA O. COYLE

Disclaimer

Hi, Valuable Reader.

Before you dive into "Expecting Excellence in Parenting," allow me to share some key phrases with you before you start your trip through its pages. This book is a labor of love that came about as a result of my own parenting experiences as well as my strong desire to encourage and uplift other people. However it's crucial to keep in mind that I am not a certified expert, and the guidance and insights offered on these pages are derived from my own experiences and study.

A family's needs may vary, and parenting is a messy, wonderful, and even plain crazy adventure. Even though I put my all into writing this book, I urge you to approach the material with an open mind and a readiness to modify it to fit your own particular set of circumstances. Never forget that you are the family's expert and that you ultimately know what is best for your kids.

Furthermore, please remember that none of the material in this book should be interpreted as professional advice; rather, it is meant mainly for general informative reasons. I strongly advise you to speak with a licensed healthcare provider or parenting specialist if you have specific worries about your child's health, development, or well-being. They can provide individualized advice that is catered to your particular requirements.

Lastly, I just wanted to say thank you so much for coming on this adventure with me. Being a parent is one of the most wonderful experiences in life, but it's also a tumultuous trip. My goal is that this book will enable you to provide a loving, caring, and satisfying environment for your family and that it will act as a source of inspiration, support, and encouragement as you traverse the highs and lows of motherhood.

Warm regards,

Patricia O. Coyle

Contents

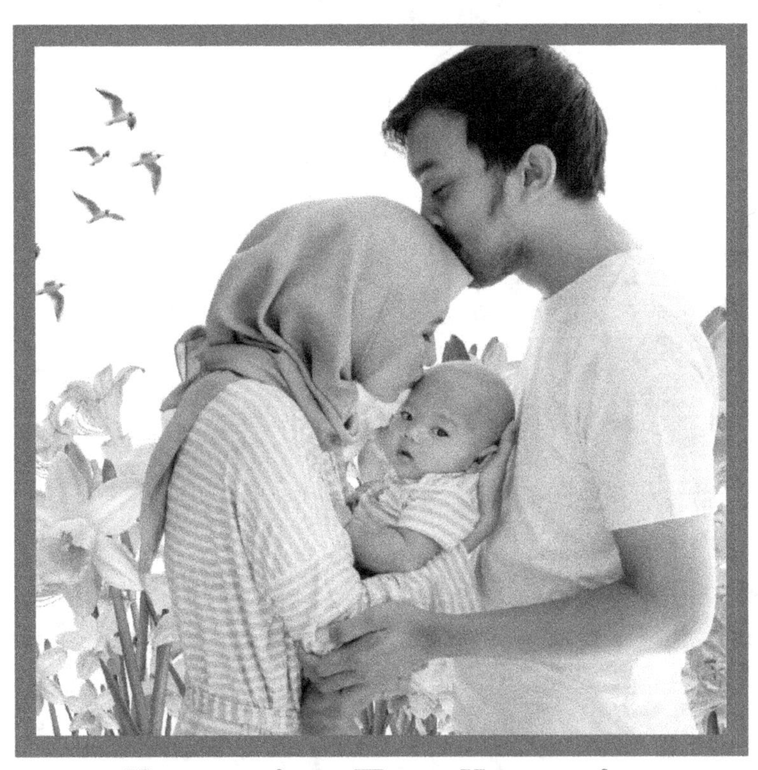

Expecting Excellence in Parenting

Introduction

The amazing adventure of motherhood starts with the quiet expectation of a newborn's first cry, in the gentle embrace of a parent's loving arms. Motherhood is a journey full of unending love, unknown obstacles, and the unwavering quest for perfection. Welcome to "Expecting Excellence in Parenting," where you will find inspiration to develop your child's potential and create relationships that will last a lifetime on every page.

Picture yourself holding your adorable baby and feeling awestruck at the wonder of life as it happens right in front of your eyes. You are overcome with amazement and wonder at that brief time, but you are also deeply responsible for creating a future full of hope and opportunity. This is the beginning of your journey, a journey filled with learning, development, and an unshakable dedication to encouraging excellence in all facets of motherhood.

However, what does it mean to demand parental excellence? It's about creating a higher standard, one based on love, compassion, and an unrelenting commitment to fostering your child's physical, emotional, and intellectual well-being. It goes beyond just meeting your child's fundamental requirements or following social conventions. It all comes down to providing an atmosphere in which your kid may grow, develop, and realize their greatest potential.

Before we go out on this life-changing adventure together, let's take a moment to consider how important it is to demand greatness from our parents. It's about realizing that every kid is a unique and priceless gift, full of individual abilities, interests, and aspirations. It is about accepting the sacred trust that has been placed in our hands as parents and devoting our whole selves to the enormous responsibility of mentoring, encouraging, and enabling our kids to reach their full potential.

This book is a veritable gold mine of knowledge, techniques, and useful advice that will enable you to face the challenges of motherhood with self-assurance, grace, and purpose. We will discuss the many delights and difficulties that come with each stage of your child's growth, from the early days of pregnancy and infancy to the turbulent terrain of toddlerhood and beyond.

Never fear, though, there will be setbacks and difficulties along the way. Motherhood is an emotional rollercoaster that requires unflinching patience, endurance, and a good dose of humor to weather the storm. From sleepless nights and teething troubles to temper tantrums and adolescent rebellion, motherhood is a rollercoaster journey. However, it is exactly by taking on these difficulties that we as parents have the chance to develop, adapt, and learn.

We shall discover the fundamental ideas and methods that serve as the cornerstone for anticipating superior parenting as we go further into the core of motherhood. We will examine the crucial role that parental influence plays in determining the course of our children's lives, from creating safe attachments and encouraging sound sleeping practices to imparting ideals of empathy, resilience, and self-discipline.

We will also explore the deep emotional journey of parenthood, which goes beyond the pragmatic aspects of raising a child. This includes the pride that fills your heart as you watch them take their first steps, and the sadness that comes with saying goodbye to them for the first time. These are the times of love, connection, and deep appreciation for the honor of leading another person's soul on their life's journey; these are the moments that epitomize fatherhood.

Thus, my dear reader, I want you to be open-minded and receptive to the many opportunities that present themselves as you set out on this incredible journey of anticipating perfection in parenting. Accept the difficulties, celebrate the successes, and treasure every minute you have with your kid. It is in these moments that parenting resides, the unbreakable relationship between a parent and child, built in love, nourished with care and intended to last a lifetime.

It's your adventure now. Let's start the adventure of expecting exceptional parenting.

Chapter *1*

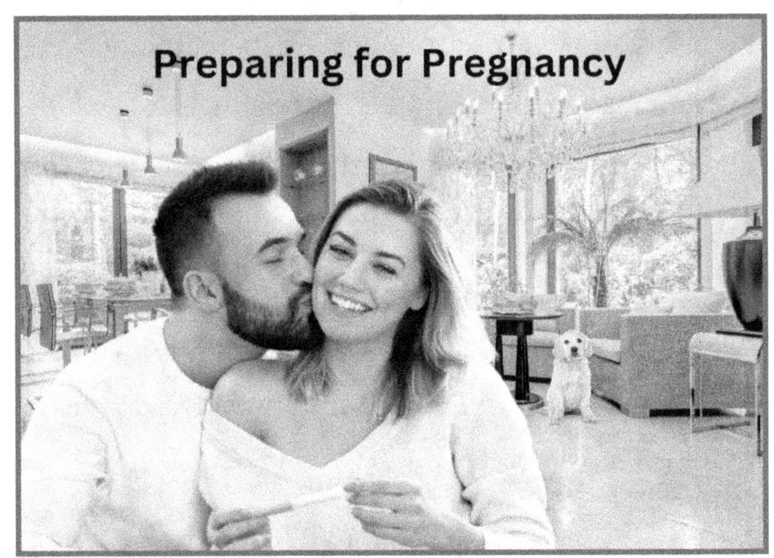

Chapter 1

Preparing for Pregnancy

Being ready both physically and emotionally for pregnancy is a thrilling and life-changing experience. Setting off on the journey to become a parent is a time of hope, excitement, and cautious preparation. A deliberate and aware attitude to this stage of life is crucial for a safe and fruitful pregnancy.

Setting your general health and well-being as a top priority is one of the first stages in getting ready for pregnancy. This involves choosing a balanced diet, keeping a healthy weight, and participating in regular exercise.

Fertility and reproductive health are supported by a balanced diet full of fruits, vegetables, whole grains, and lean meats, which supply vital nutrients. Regular exercise also aids in promoting general vitality, lowering stress levels, and improving circulation, all of which are critical aspects of body readiness for pregnancy.

It's critical to treat any underlying medical issues that may affect fertility or pregnancy outcomes in addition to concentrating on physical health. This might include making an appointment for a preconception check-up where you can talk to your doctor about your health history, get the tests you need, and get tailored advice on how to improve your health before becoming pregnant.

Resolving any pre-existing health issues, such as thyroid abnormalities, hypertension, or diabetes, might reduce the likelihood of difficulties and dangers during pregnancy.

Individuals and couples should think about any known genetic disorders that might affect pregnancy, as well as the medical history of their family. For those who have a family history of chromosomal abnormalities, genetic illnesses, or hereditary ailments, genetic counseling may be advised. Informed choices on family planning and prenatal care may be made by people with the assistance of genetic testing and counseling, which can provide vital information regarding possible dangers.

Examining your menstrual cycle and determining your viable window are essential components of getting ready for motherhood. Tracking your menstrual cycle and ovulation might help you determine the best period for conception. You may improve your chances of becoming pregnant by using tools like fertility monitoring apps or ovulation prediction kits to help you figure out when you're most likely to ovulate.

When getting ready for pregnancy, emotional preparedness is just as crucial. Being a parent is a transformative experience that requires a solid base of emotional support and perseverance. Give your expectations, worries, and wishes for parenting some thought. Talk honestly about your thoughts with your spouse and other family members. If necessary, get help from dependable friends, relatives, or mental health specialists.

In addition to physical and mental preparation, financial planning is a vital element of preparing for pregnancy. Costs associated with being a parent include those related to prenatal care, delivery, and daycare. Spend some time evaluating your present financial status, making a budget, and arranging for any supplementary costs related to beginning or growing a family.

As you get ready for the financial demands of parenting, think about things like health insurance coverage, maternity leave regulations, and daycare alternatives.

Establishing a supportive atmosphere that promotes conception and successful pregnancy outcomes is another essential component of getting ready for motherhood. This may require adopting lifestyle alterations such as lowering exposure to environmental pollutants, stopping smoking, limiting alcohol use, and avoiding recreational drugs.

Fostering a loving and stress-free atmosphere may also have a favorable effect on general well-being and fertility.

Lastly, it's critical to foster candid communication and teamwork with your spouse over the whole pregnancy preparation process. Being a parent is a collaborative endeavor that calls for dedication, understanding, and support from both sides.

Talk about your expectations, aspirations, and wishes for motherhood with someone, and together come up with a strategy that reflects your common values and objectives.

Consulting with a Healthcare Provider

Making an appointment for a preconception visit with a healthcare professional is an essential first step in getting ready for pregnancy. People may review their medical history, talk about their goals to get pregnant and receive tailored advice on how to best prepare their health for conception at this session.

The medical professional may do a physical examination, evaluate the patient's present state of health, and answer any queries or worries about conception, and pregnancy care.

Reaching a Healthy Weight: Fertility and the success of pregnancy depend on maintaining a healthy weight. Overweight or underweight people may have trouble becoming pregnant and run a higher risk of having problems during pregnancy. Achieving a body mass index (BMI) within the suggested range for your height and build is crucial before trying to conceive. Developing a customized strategy for achieving and maintaining a healthy weight via a mix of balanced eating, consistent exercise, and lifestyle changes may be facilitated by working with a medical professional or registered dietitian.

Handling Chronic Health Problems: Fertility and pregnancy outcomes may be impacted by chronic health problems such as diabetes, hypertension, thyroid issues, and autoimmune illnesses. It's essential to make sure these problems are well-managed and under control before becoming pregnant.

To maximize health, this may include modifying lifestyle choices, monitoring blood pressure or blood sugar levels, and modifying prescription schedules.

Healthcare professionals may provide advice on how to minimize risks to the mother and unborn child and manage chronic health concerns throughout pregnancy.

Developing Healthy Lifestyle Practices: Fertility and pregnancy health are significantly impacted by the adoption of healthy lifestyle practices. When considering pregnancy, people should concentrate on forming routines that promote general well-being, such as:

Consuming a well-balanced diet full of whole grains, fruits, vegetables, lean meats, and healthy fats provides vital nutrients for fetal growth and fertility. Frequent physical exercise to enhance general fitness, lower stress, and maintain a healthy weight.

As advised by healthcare professionals, try to get in at least 30 minutes of moderate-intensity activity most days of the week. Sleeping enough is important for immune system performance, hormone balance, and general wellness. To encourage good sleeping habits, aim for 7-9 hours of quality sleep each night and create a regular sleep regimen.

Using mindfulness exercises, relaxation methods, and stress-relieving hobbies like yoga, meditation, or outdoor time to manage stress. Prioritizing stress management before conception is crucial since prolonged stress may impair fertility and raise the chance of pregnancy problems.

Taking Prenatal Vitamins: Preconception health and fitness are greatly aided by the use of prenatal vitamins. Important minerals including folic acid, iron, calcium, and vitamin D are included in these supplements, which are essential for maintaining the health of both the mother and the fetus throughout pregnancy.

Particularly folic acid has a significant role in lowering the chance of neural tube abnormalities in the growing child; thus, it is advised that women begin taking a daily prenatal vitamin containing 400 micrograms or more of folic acid before conception and continue doing so for the duration of their pregnancy.

Understanding Reproductive Health: A variety of variables affect an individual's capacity to conceive and carry a baby to term, and reproductive health is not only about fertility. People should have a thorough awareness of all aspects of their reproductive health, including the regularity of their menstrual cycle, the patterns of ovulation, and any underlying medical disorders that may have an impact on fertility or conception.

Menstrual cycle tracking and fertility sign monitoring may provide important insights into reproductive health and assist in identifying any problems that may need further assessment by a medical professional.

Evaluating Environmental Exposures: Reproductive health and fertility may be impacted by environmental variables. People should be aware of any environmental exposures, such as exposure to chemicals, poisons, pollutants, and environmental dangers, that may have an impact on fertility.

Reducing environmental exposure to toxic chemicals at work and home may enhance preconception health and safeguard fertility. This might include altering one's way of life, donning safety gear, and, if required, pushing for better living and working conditions.

Accepting Holistic well-being: Holistic well-being, which includes mental, emotional, and physical health, is what is meant by preconception health, which goes beyond physical well-being. Developing emotional resilience, stress management techniques and supportive connections are all part of putting holistic wellbeing first. Preconception health may be improved and people can be better prepared for the emotional roller coaster of pregnancy and motherhood by partaking in activities that encourage self-care, relaxation, and emotional balance, such as mindfulness exercises, journaling, or counseling.

Encouraging Male Preconception Health: Although female reproductive health receives a lot of attention when it comes to preconception health, male preconception health should also be prioritized.

Fertility and pregnancy outcomes are influenced by male variables; thus, enhancing male preconception health may increase the odds of conception and promote a healthy pregnancy. Men should put their preconception of health first by leading healthy lives, abstaining from drugs, and taking care of any underlying medical issues that could have an impact on fertility.

Understanding Fertility and Conception

Fertility and conception are complex processes that depend on several variables, including menstrual cycles, ovulation, timing of sexual activity, and reproductive health. It's crucial for people and couples who are planning a pregnancy or attempting to conceive to fully comprehend these ideas.

1. **Menstrual Cycle and Ovulation:** A crucial component of female fertility and reproductive health is the menstrual cycle. It is controlled by variations in hormone levels in the body and usually lasts for 28 days, however individual cycles may be longer or shorter. Knowing the stages of the menstrual cycle, menstruation, follicular phase, ovulation, and luteal phase, is essential to understanding it.

- **Menstruation:** The removal of the uterine lining during menstruation causes vaginal bleeding and signifies the start of the monthly cycle. Most times, it takes three to seven days.

- **Follicular Phase:** Ovulation marks the end of the follicular phase, which starts on the first day of menstruation. To prepare for a possible pregnancy, the uterine lining thickens and follicles in the ovaries develop during this period.

- **Ovulation:** On average, a 28-day cycle's ovulation takes place between days 11 and 21 of the menstrual cycle. The menstrual cycle's most fertile time is signaled by the release of a mature egg from one of the ovaries.

- **Luteal Phase:** The luteal phase, which lasts until the beginning of the subsequent menstrual cycle, starts after ovulation. In this stage, the broken follicle develops into the corpus luteum, a tissue that, in the event of a pregnancy, releases progesterone to nourish the lining of the uterus.

2. Establishing the Fertile Window: The window of opportunity during which conception is most likely to occur is known as the fertile window. It usually lasts for a few days both before and on the actual day of ovulation. It is essential to know the fertile window to schedule sexual activity in a way that maximizes the likelihood of pregnancy.

- **Basal Body Temperature (BBT):** Taking your body's temperature first thing in the morning and charting it is the process of tracking basal body temperature. The viable window may be determined with the assistance of a minor rise in basal body temperature, which signifies the occurrence of ovulation.

- **Changes in Cervical Mucus:** Throughout the menstrual cycle, variations in the texture and consistency of cervical mucus might provide information regarding fertility. Cervical mucus usually turns clear, slick, and elastic as ovulation draws near, akin to egg whites.

- **Ovulation Predictor Kits (OPKs):** OPKs measure the spike in luteinizing hormone (LH) that occurs just before ovulation. People may determine when ovulation is likely to happen and when is the best time to have sex by utilizing an OPK.

3. Appropriate Timing and Frequency of Intercourse: During the fertile window, frequent, unprotected sexual activity increases the likelihood of pregnancy. The objective of scheduling sexual activity is to make sure that sperm are present in the reproductive canal at the time of ovulation, however, there is no one-size-fits-all method.

- **Every one to two days:** During the fertile window, experts usually advise having intercourse every one to two days to maximize the chances of conceiving. By guaranteeing that sperm are in the reproductive canal both before and during ovulation, this frequency raises the possibility of conception.

- **Setting Ovulation Day as a Priority:** While frequent sexual activity throughout the fertile window is excellent, setting Ovulation Day as a Priority might further boost the likelihood of pregnancy. Sperm can fertilize the egg most effectively if they time their sexual activity around the time of ovulation.

4. Understanding Male Fertility: Male variables are important in conception as well; fertility is not only a feminine problem. It is important to understand the variables that affect sperm function, quality, and production to comprehend male fertility.

- **Sperm Health:** Healthy sperm are essential for pregnancy and fertility. The health of sperm may be influenced by several factors, including age, underlying medical disorders (such as varicocele or hormone imbalances), environmental exposures (like heat, radiation, or pollutants), and lifestyle choices (including smoking, binge drinking, and drug use).
- **Semen Analysis:** This diagnostic test counts the number of sperm and assesses their motility (movement), morphology (shape), and other characteristics. It assists in evaluating male fertility and locating any possible problems that can impede pregnancy.

- **Improving Male Fertility:** Men may improve their fertility by leading healthy lifestyles, abstaining from drugs and alcohol, and taking care of any underlying medical issues. This includes keeping a healthy weight, eating a balanced diet, exercising often, protecting the genital region from excessive heat exposure, and using safe sexual practices to prevent STDs.

Chapter 2

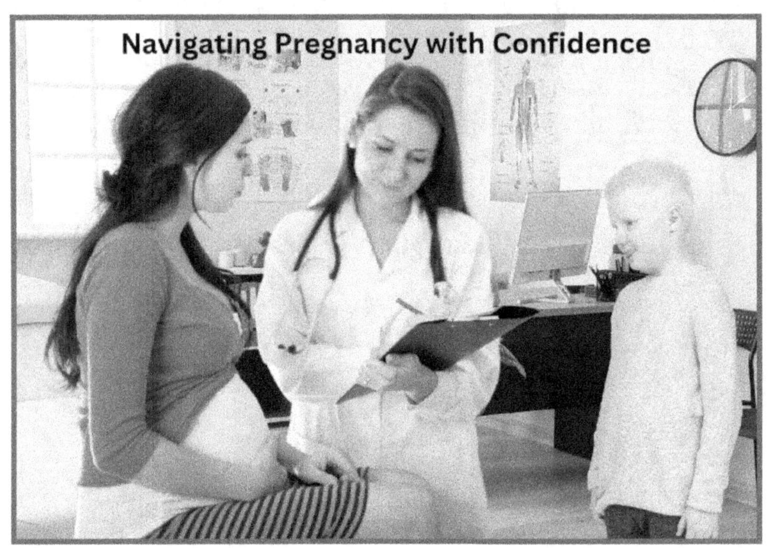

Navigating Pregnancy with Confidence

Being a confident pregnant woman means accepting the journey with optimism, education, and proactive self-care techniques. The following are some essential pointers to help you confidently handle pregnancy:

Educate Yourself: Invest some time in learning about pregnancy, labor, and the post-partum period. To learn about the changes and difficulties of pregnancy, take prenatal courses, read credible books and articles, and speak with medical professionals.

Pay Attention to Your Body: Throughout your pregnancy, pay attention to your body's clues and messages. To promote both your health and the health of your unborn child, take breaks when necessary, drink enough water, and eat a healthy diet.

Talk Honestly: Keep lines of communication open and honest with your medical professional. Throughout your prenatal care experience, voice any concerns or inquiries you may have and act as an advocate for your needs and preferences.

Keep Moving: Take frequent, safe, and stage-appropriate physical exercise during your pregnancy. You may improve your mood, vitality, and general well-being by engaging in activities like swimming, walking, prenatal yoga, and light stretching.

Seek Support: Assemble a network of family, friends, and medical professionals who are willing to lend a hand when necessary and who can provide encouragement, direction, and support. In trying circumstances, don't be afraid to ask for assistance or seek out emotional support.

Practice Self-Care: Give self-care activities that support emotional health, stress relief, and relaxation top priority. Spend time relaxing, engaging in enjoyable hobbies, and practicing mindfulness and relaxation methods.

Get Ready for Delivery: Learn about alternatives for childbirth, how to handle discomfort and the labor and delivery process. Create a birth plan that details your choices for delivery and labor, and talk to your birth team and healthcare provider about it.

Remain Upbeat: Remain upbeat and concentrate on the happiness and excitement of having your kid. Throughout your pregnancy, surround yourself with people who will support and encourage you, as well as positive thoughts and affirmations.

Nutrition and Prenatal Care

A good pregnancy journey must include prenatal care and nutrition since they provide the groundwork for the growing baby's health as well as the pregnant parent's. Prioritizing prenatal care and nutrition may help maintain optimum mother health, fetal growth and development, and excellent pregnancy outcomes from the early stages of pregnancy through birthing and beyond.

Comprehensive Prenatal Care: Throughout pregnancy, prospective parents and their unborn child's health are monitored by healthcare professionals via routine physical examinations, tests, and counseling.

A variety of services are included in comprehensive prenatal care with the goals of advancing the mother's health, identifying and treating pregnancy-related issues, and fostering the growth and development of the fetus.

Early Prenatal Visits: Ideally, the first prenatal visit takes place in the first trimester of pregnancy. To create a customized treatment plan for the pregnancy, medical professionals do a comprehensive review of the patient's medical history, a physical examination, and baseline evaluations during this first appointment.

Frequent Check-ups: Expectant parents see their healthcare providers for routine prenatal check-ups throughout their pregnancy. These appointments are typically arranged every 4-6 weeks during the first two trimesters and increasingly often as the pregnancy goes on.

Healthcare professionals check the health of the mother and fetus at these visits, evaluate growth and development, do standard screenings and tests, and provide advice on any pregnancy-related problems.

Screenings and Tests: To evaluate the health of the mother and look for any possible pregnancy issues, prenatal care involves several screenings and tests. Blood tests, ultrasound scans, genetic screening, glucose tolerance testing for gestational diabetes, and other specialist tests depending on a patient's unique risk factors and medical history may be part of these screenings.

Prenatal care visits provide chances for information, guidance, and support on a range of topics related to pregnancy, labor, and postpartum care. Healthcare professionals may provide advice on parenting styles, breastfeeding, prenatal vitamins, exercise, labor and delivery alternatives, and diet.

They also answer any questions or worries the expecting parent may have and provide advice on how to deal with the difficulties and discomforts that come with being pregnant.

Optimizing Prenatal Nutrition: To support the health of the mother, the growth and development of the fetus, and the success of the pregnancy as a whole, adequate nutrition is essential throughout pregnancy.

An adequate diet that is rich in nutrients and well-balanced supplies vital vitamins, minerals, protein, carbs, fats, and calories that are needed for both the health and well-being of the developing child and the expecting mother.

Important Nutrients for Pregnancy: To promote fetal growth and development, pregnant women need to consume more nutrients than non-pregnant people do. Iron, calcium, vitamin D, omega-3 fatty acids, protein, folic acid, and vitamin D are important nutrients during pregnancy. The formation of the neural tube, the synthesis of red blood cells, bone health, immunological function, and brain development are all dependent on these nutrients.

Balanced Diet: Throughout pregnancy, a healthy diet should consist of a range of nutrient-dense foods from all food categories, such as whole grains, fruits, vegetables, lean meats, dairy products, and healthy fats. Consuming a wide variety of meals improves overall maternal and fetal health and helps guarantee appropriate intake of vital nutrients.

Hydration: Maintaining enough fluid intake during pregnancy is crucial for maintaining the mother's blood flow, the baby's absorption of nutrients, and the levels of amniotic fluid. Drinking plenty of water throughout the day and avoiding sugary and caffeinated drinks is advised for pregnant women. Drinking enough water may help avoid dehydration, constipation, UTIs, and other pregnancy-related issues.

Supplementation: To guarantee appropriate consumption of essential nutrients during pregnancy and to address nutritional gaps, prenatal vitamins are advised in addition to a balanced diet. Healthcare professionals usually prescribe or suggest prenatal vitamins that include folic acid, iron, calcium, vitamin D, and other vital nutrients to promote the health of both the mother and the fetus.

Following a doctor's instructions and taking prenatal vitamins will assist ensure the best possible result for your unborn child and help avoid nutritional deficits.

Food Safety: To lower the risk of foodborne infections, which may endanger the health of both the mother and the fetus, pregnant women should be aware of the regulations governing food safety. To reduce the risk of foodborne infections and pollutants, it is advised to avoid several high-risk foods, such as unpasteurized dairy products, raw or undercooked meats and seafood, deli meats, and high-mercury fish.

Food Aversions and Cravings: Hormones related to pregnancy may cause changes in how people perceive taste and scent, which may result in food aversions or cravings. It is possible to fulfill cravings and aversions while meeting nutritional demands by paying attention to your body's signals and preferences, including a range of nutrient-rich foods in your diet, and indulging in urges in moderation.

Food Allergies and Intolerances: To achieve nutritional requirements and prevent possible allergens or triggers, it is important to pay close attention to dietary choices while managing food allergies or intolerances during pregnancy.

A licensed dietitian or healthcare professional should collaborate with people who have food allergies or intolerances to create a safe and nourishing meal plan that satisfies their dietary requirements.

Diabetes during pregnancy: Diabetes during pregnancy is a kind of diabetes that has to be carefully managed with food, exercise, and, in some situations, medication. For those with gestational diabetes, maintaining a balanced diet full of fiber, lean proteins, complex carbs, and healthy fats will help control blood sugar levels and promote the best possible pregnancy outcomes.

Guidelines for Weight Increase: Based on pre-pregnancy body mass index (BMI), the Institute of Medicine (IOM) offers guidelines for gestational weight increase.

It is generally suggested that pregnant women with normal pre-pregnancy BMIs (18.5-24.9) gain 25–35 pounds; however, recommended ranges may vary for those with underweight or overweight/obese BMI categories.

Individualized Approach: Depending on a person's pre-pregnancy BMI, dietary state, and underlying medical issues, different weight gain rates may be advised. Healthcare professionals collaborate with pregnant parents to create individualized weight gain targets and track their progress throughout the pregnancy.

Monitoring Weight increase: During prenatal visits, healthcare professionals keep a close eye on patients' weight increase to make sure it is by personalized objectives and advised guidelines.

Excessive or rapid weight gain may be a sign of preeclampsia, gestational diabetes, or fetal macrosomia (high birth weight), which calls for more testing and care.

Unique Dietary Considerations

To maximize mother and fetal health and meet particular nutritional demands, several pregnancy-related situations or conditions may call for unique dietary considerations. Pregnancy-related situations such as:

Multiple Gestation: To support the growth and development of multiple fetuses, individuals carrying twins, triplets, or higher-order multiples have special dietary needs. To fulfill the demands of multiple pregnancies, healthcare practitioners may suggest consuming more calories, protein, and certain minerals like calcium and iron.

Vegan or Vegetarian Diets: When properly designed to provide sufficient consumption of vital minerals including zinc, iron, calcium, vitamin B12, omega-3 fatty acids, and protein, vegan and vegetarian diets may coexist with a healthy pregnancy. A certified dietitian or healthcare professional should be consulted by pregnant women who follow vegetarian or vegan diets to create a nutritionally balanced meal plan and to discuss supplementation if necessary to fulfill their increased nutrient demands during pregnancy.

Personal Preferences: During pregnancy, dietary habits and meal choices are influenced by an individual's likes, aversions, and preferences. Expectant parents should prioritize satisfying their child's nutritional demands for a successful pregnancy and feel empowered to make educated choices about their food preferences.

Flexibility and Adaptability: Dietary requirements and preferences may alter throughout a pregnancy, which is a period of transition and change. Prenatal nutrition and well-being may be continuously supported by addressing concerns, navigating dietary problems, and keeping lines of communication open and flexible with healthcare practitioners.

Handling Typical Pregnancy Pains

While being pregnant is an amazing experience full of excitement and expectation, the body goes through significant changes to support the developing baby, which may also cause several discomforts and difficulties.

Expectant parents may go through this trip with more comfort and confidence if they are aware of and adept at treating certain typical pregnancy discomforts.

1. **Nausea and vomiting (morning sickness):** Among the most frequent symptoms of pregnancy, especially in the first trimester, are nausea and vomiting (morning sickness). Even though morning

sickness may be difficult to deal with, there are a few ways to manage its symptoms:

Eat Small, Often: Eating small, frequent meals throughout the day may help control blood sugar levels and reduce nausea. Choose simple, easily digested items like rice, bread, crackers, or bananas.

Keep Yourself Hydrated: Drink plenty of water, ginger ale, herbal teas, or electrolyte-rich drinks to remain hydrated since dehydration may worsen nausea. Some people find that nibbling on ginger candies or sipping ginger tea helps them feel better.

Steer clear of trigger foods: Certain foods and scents might cause motion sickness and vomiting. Choose moderate, non-greasy, and easier-on-the-tummy meals instead of ones that worsen your symptoms.

Try Acupressure Bands: Some people find that applying pressure to certain acupressure spots on the wrist using acupressure bracelets may help reduce nausea. Pharmacies and internet merchants sell these bands.

Think About Medications: To alleviate severe morning sickness, doctors may recommend anti-nausea drugs like Zofran (ondansetron) or Diclegis (doxylamine succinate and pyridoxine hydrochloride). A healthcare professional should always be consulted before taking any medicine while pregnant.

2. Heartburn and Indigestion: These two pregnancy discomforts are frequent, especially in the latter stages when the expanding uterus presses on the stomach. To properly treat indigestion and heartburn, take into account the following tactics:

Eat Smaller Meals: Eating more often and in smaller portions will help reduce the symptoms of heartburn and avoid overflowing the stomach.

Choose to eat smaller meals instead of larger ones just before bed.

Steer Clear of Trigger Foods and Beverages: These include chocolate, coffee, citrus fruits, tomatoes, spicy meals, and carbonated drinks. They may also cause indigestion and heartburn. To lessen symptoms, identify and stay away from items that trigger you.

Stay Upright After Eating: You may help avoid heartburn by keeping your stomach acid from refluxing into your esophagus by staying upright for at least thirty minutes after eating. Recessing or lying down just after eating is not advised.

Use Cushions for Support: Keeping your head and chest up as you sleep, elevating the head of your bed with cushions, or placing a wedge-shaped pillow beneath your upper torso might help lessen the sensations of heartburn at night.

Think About Antacids: An antacid that may be purchased over-the-counter, such as Maalox, Rolaids, or Tums, can provide momentary relief from acid reflux and heartburn. But before using antacids, see a doctor, particularly if you have any other medical concerns or are on other drugs.

3. Backache and Pelvic Pain: These two frequent pregnancy discomforts are experienced by many, especially in the latter stages as the body adapts to the increased weight and posture changes. Take into consideration the following tactics for efficient management of pelvic pain and backache:

Maintain Excellent Posture: Keeping your back and pelvis from being overworked may be achieved by maintaining excellent posture. Maintain an upright posture, stand with your shoulders back and your pelvis tucked, and try not to slouch or arch your back too much.

Employ Good Body Mechanics: To lessen the pressure on your back and pelvis, bend at the knees and hips rather than at the waist while lifting items or bending over. Steer clear of heavy lifting and ask for assistance with jobs that need a lot of effort.

Remain Active: Regular exercise helps build the muscles that support the pelvis and back, which lowers the chance of pain and discomfort. To increase muscle tone and flexibility, think about doing mild workouts like swimming, walking, prenatal yoga, or pelvic floor exercises (Kegels).

Apply Heat or Cold treatment: Reducing inflammation and easing discomfort in the afflicted regions may be achieved by applying heat or cold treatment. For back pain, use a heating pad, warm compress, or hot water bottle; for pelvic discomfort, use an ice pack or cold pack on the pelvis.

Employ Supportive Devices: By adding extra support to the abdomen and pelvis, belly bands, or pelvic support garments help ease the pressure on the lower back and pelvic joints. Seek advice from a physical therapist or healthcare professional on suitable assistive technology.

4. Fatigue and Sleep disturbances: During the first and third trimesters of pregnancy, fatigue, and sleep disturbances are prevalent symptoms. Take into consideration the following tactics to control weariness and enhance the quality of your sleep:

Prioritize Rest: Pay attention to your body's signals and make time for relaxation when necessary. To tell your body when it's time to wind down, take short naps throughout the day, engage in relaxation exercises like deep breathing or meditation, and create a nighttime routine.

Ensure a Comfortable Sleep Environment: Keep your bedroom cold, dark, and quiet to create a suitable sleeping environment. To reduce pain and encourage better sleep posture, use supportive pillows. If you need more support, think about using a pregnant pillow.

Maintain appropriate Sleep Hygiene: To enhance the quality of your sleep, maintain appropriate sleep hygiene practices. To manage your body's internal clock, avoid stimulants like coffee and screen time before bed, and create a regular sleep pattern.

Keep Yourself Active: Getting regular exercise throughout the day may help lower weariness and enhance the quality of your sleep. Try to get some moderate activity, like swimming, walking, or prenatal fitness courses, but stay away from intense exertion just before bed.

Seek Support: When you're feeling worn out or overburdened, don't be afraid to approach your spouse, family, or friends for assistance. Assign responsibilities, give self-care priority, and express your requirements to others to make sure you get the pregnancy support you need.

5. Swelling and Fluid Retention: Often affecting the hands, feet, ankles, and legs, swelling and fluid retention, or edema, are frequent symptoms of pregnancy.

While some edema is typical during pregnancy, sudden or excessive swelling should be checked by a healthcare professional since it may suggest possible concerns like preeclampsia. To control edema and fluid retention:

Keep Yourself Hydrated: This is crucial and should not be understated. Reducing fluid retention and preventing dehydration may both be achieved by drinking plenty of water. Try to consume 8 to 10 glasses of water a day or more, and avoid overindulging in salty or caffeinated meals since they may also lead to fluid retention.

Elevate Your Legs: Whenever feasible, raise your legs above the level of your heart to aid in circulation and lessen edema in your lower limbs. When sitting or lying down, raise your legs using cushions, and try not to stay still for extended periods.

Put on Comfortable Shoes: Opt for supportive, comfy shoes with low heels and enough wiggle space to accommodate swelling. To accommodate variations in foot size, use sandals or shoes with Velcro straps that are adjustable instead of socks or shoes that are too tight and impede circulation.

Exercise Gently: Walking, swimming, or prenatal yoga are examples of mild workouts that may assist improve circulation and minimize edema. Steer clear of high-impact exercises that might aggravate swelling or pain, and pay attention to your body's signals to prevent exerting yourself too much.

Wear Compression Garments: Socks or compression stockings may aid with circulation and minimize foot and leg edema. When standing or sitting for extended periods, use compression clothing throughout the day. At night, take them off to give your legs a chance to recover.

6. Emotional Changes and Stress: A pregnant woman's body goes through a lot of emotional and psychological changes, which are often accompanied by stress, elevated anxiety, and mood swings. To minimize stress and handle emotional shifts during pregnancy:

Practice Self-Care: Give self-care activities that support emotional health, stress relief, and relaxation top priority. Take part in things you love doing, including reading, watching TV, going on walks in the park, or learning mindfulness and meditation methods.

Seek Support: For emotional support and motivation, reach out to your spouse, your family, your friends, or support organizations. During stressful or uncertain times, confiding in trustworthy people about your thoughts and emotions may provide validation, solace, and confidence.

Interact with Your Healthcare Physician: Don't be afraid to talk to your healthcare physician about your emotional worries and anxieties. They may provide direction, encouragement, and tools to aid with stress management and take care of any underlying mental health conditions like depression or anxiety.

Practice Relaxation methods: To promote relaxation and lower stress levels, including relaxation methods like progressive muscle relaxation, guided imagery, and deep breathing exercises into your daily routine. Regular use of these methods may help reduce stress and anxiety by calming the body and mind.

Remain Active: Engaging in regular physical exercise releases endorphins, which are the body's natural feel-good chemicals that may help lower stress and elevate mood. Walk, swim, or practice prenatal yoga as a mild kind of exercise to improve your mood and general health.

When to Consult a Doctor

While many of the symptoms of pregnancy are common and anticipated, some could point to a more severe underlying issue that needs to be treated right away. If a pregnant woman has any of the following symptoms, she should speak with her doctor:

1. Severe or Persistent Vomiting and Nausea: Hyperemesis gravidarum is a severe kind of morning sickness that might need medical attention. It is characterized by persistent vomiting, dehydration, nausea, and weight loss.

2. Vaginal Bleeding: To rule out problems like miscarriage or an ectopic pregnancy, any vaginal bleeding that occurs during pregnancy, particularly in the first trimester, should be investigated by a healthcare professional.

3. Severe Abdomen Pain: It is important to get immediate medical attention if you have severe or ongoing abdomen pain, cramps, or pelvic pressure since these may be signs of issues such as premature labor, placental abruption, or preeclampsia.

4. Sudden Swelling or Fluid Retention: Sudden weight gain, changes in eyesight, or sudden or severe swelling of the hands, feet, or face might all be indicators of preeclampsia, and should be treated as soon as possible.

5. Reduced Fetal Movement: Fetal distress should be reported right away to a healthcare professional if there is a decrease in fetal movement or if there are changes in the patterns of fetal activity.

6. Infection Warning Signs: Feelings like the flu, persistent vomiting or diarrhea, fever, chills, and other symptoms may point to an infection that needs to be treated by a doctor.

Chapter 3

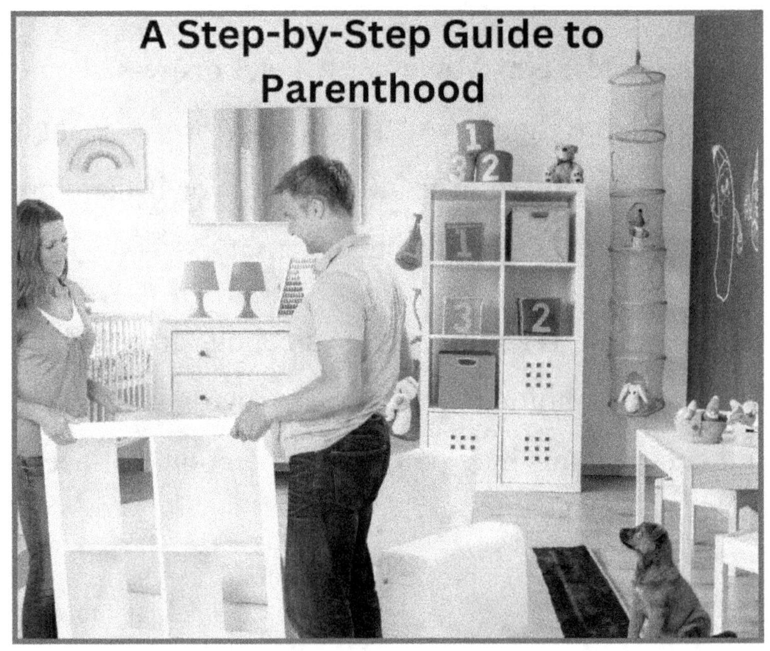

Chapter 3

Step-by-Step Guide to Parenthood

Being a parent is a life-changing experience full of happiness, difficulties, and limitless learning possibilities. Here is a step-by-step approach to assist you enter parenthood with grace and confidence:

Planning and Preparation: Spend some time learning about pregnancy, labor, and parenting to better prepare yourself for becoming a parent. Take prenatal seminars, read credible books and articles, and ask medical experts and seasoned parents for assistance.

Talk to your spouse or other support system about your aspirations, worries, and expectations about being a parent. Create a common future vision and a channel of open communication for your family.

Prenatal Care and Health: Throughout your pregnancy, put your health and well-being first by eating a balanced diet, drinking lots of water, exercising often, getting enough rest, and visiting prenatal checkups regularly.

To promote a healthy pregnancy and the best possible fetal growth, heed the advice of your healthcare practitioner about prenatal vitamins, screenings, and testing.

Preparing for Childbirth: Learn as much as you can about giving birth, including the many alternatives, how to handle discomfort, and how to attend courses. Create a birth plan that lists your goals and preferences for the labor and delivery process. Stuff a hospital bag with necessities for you and your companion, including clothes, toiletries, food, and comfort things.

Welcoming Your New Baby: Get your house ready for your baby's birth by establishing a nursery, baby-proofing your rooms, and preparing a supply closet full of necessities like clothes, diapers, wipes, and feeding equipment. Establish a network of family, friends, and medical experts to help you cope with the responsibilities of caring for a baby and support you throughout the postpartum time.

Attachment & Bonding: Create a strong emotional connection with your infant via gentle touch, nursing, bottle feeding, and skin-to-skin contact. You should establish a strong attachment link with your infant and react quickly to their indications. Take part in activities like singing, reading, chatting, and playing with your infant that foster a strong link between parents and children. Establish a solid foundation of love, trust, and kinship that will strengthen your bond with your kids as they become older.

Managing Parenting Difficulties: Get ready for the rigors of motherhood, such as lack of sleep, feeding issues, and transitioning to your new role. Consult medical experts, parental associations, and internet forums for assistance in addressing your worries and acquiring coping mechanisms.

Make self-care a priority and give your mental, emotional, and physical health priority. Ask for assistance from others in your support system when necessary, take pauses, and be honest with your spouse about your needs and emotions.

Learning and Developing Together: Accept motherhood as an ongoing process of learning, development, and exploration. As you negotiate the ups and downs of parenthood, practice patience with both yourself and your kid. Look for educational and enrichment possibilities via community resources, parenting courses, books, and seminars. Remain inquisitive, adaptable, and receptive as you adjust to your child's changing needs and interests.

Relishing Memories and Milestones: From your baby's first grin to their first steps and beyond, cherish and mark the unique occasions and milestones of motherhood. Capture the wonder of childhood in pictures, movies, and mementos to create enduring memories.

Spend some time thinking back on your parenting path and acknowledging your successes, development, and fortitude. Savor the delight and amazement of being a parent as you see your child's growth and development.

Getting Your Home Ready for a Newcomer

Getting ready for a new baby to arrive at your house is an exciting and significant process. Establishing a secure, cozy, and supportive space is crucial to embracing your child and guaranteeing their welfare. The following crucial actions will assist you in preparing your house for your new arrival:

Essentials for a Nursery: Set aside a calm, comfortable area of your house for the nursery. When it comes to feedings and changes at night, choose a spot that is convenient for you and near to your bedroom. Stock the nursery with necessities like a changing table or dresser that can hold plenty of clothes, wipes, diaper storage, a cot or bassinet, and a cozy rocking rocker or glider for feeding and comforting your child.

To make the nursery seem cozy and peaceful for your infant, decorate it with muted hues and soft lighting. Steer clear of extra decorations and clutter that might endanger your safety.

Safety Precautions: To avoid falls and mishaps, place safety gates at the top and bottom of stairs. To stop them from toppling, fasten large furniture pieces like TVs, dressers, and bookshelves to the wall. Electrical outlets, cables, and sharp edges should all have guards and safety coverings to keep babies safe. Prevent inquisitive hands and mouths from accessing tiny items, choking dangers, and dangerous chemicals. To keep an eye on your child as they play or sleep in their nursery, use a baby monitor that has audio and video features.

Feeding and Diapering Stations: Arrange a nursing cushion for support, a side table with necessities like bottles, breast pumps, and burp cloths, and a cozy rocker or glider to create a handy and pleasant feeding station in your house.

Make sure your diapering station is well prepared with a changing table or pad, wipes, diaper rash ointment, diapers in different sizes, and a diaper pail for convenient disposal of used diapers. For hygiene, have hand sanitizer close by.

Clothes and Linens: To accommodate your baby's development, stock up on basic infant clothes items like onesies, sleepers, socks, hats, and mittens in several sizes. For your baby's crib or bassinet, spend money on breathable, soft bedding and linens.

This includes fitted sheets, blankets, swaddles, and mattress covers. Steer clear of soft toys and unsecured bedding that might suffocate a child.

Storage and Arrangement: Set aside specific spaces for the storage of necessities for the baby, including clothes, wipes, diapers, feeding supplies, toys, and linens. To keep things neat and handy, use drawers, shelves, bins, and baskets. To optimize storage space in tiny or shared living rooms, think about investing in space-saving storage solutions like hanging organizers, under-bed storage bins, and multipurpose furniture.

Baby-Friendly Environment: Provide your infant with a calm and engaging space with age-appropriate toys, books, and soft lighting and music. Give children the chance to explore and develop their senses with tactile books, fluffy toys, and vibrant mobiles.

To make your infant feel safe and at ease in their new surroundings, create a regular daily schedule and nighttime habit. Maintain regular sleeping, eating, and playing schedules to encourage healthy development.

Siblings and pets should be prepared as well. If you have older kids or pets, include them in the process and assist them in adjusting to the impending changes in the family dynamic. Invite siblings to help with the nursery setup and get everything ready for the new baby's arrival.

Gradually and kindly introduce dogs to baby products including strollers, cribs, and baby gear. To make dogs feel safe and part of the family, give them plenty of love, exercise, and supervision.

Budgeting and Financial Planning for Parenthood

Being a parent is a wonderful adventure full of love, and novel experiences, but it also entails heavy financial obligations. It's essential to budget for child-rearing expenses if you want to guarantee the health and financial security of your family. This is a thorough resource that will assist you with budgeting and financial planning as a parent:

1. Evaluate Your Present Financial Condition

- Assessing your income, spending, savings, obligations, and financial objectives is a good place to start. Assess your financial holdings, including retirement plans, savings accounts, and investments, as well as any debt you may have from credit card debt or loans.

- To ascertain your cash flow and find places where you might cut costs or reallocate money to support your expanding family, compute your monthly income and expenditures.

2. Calculate Expected Child-Related Costs

Ascertain the expected expenses related to becoming a parent, such as:

- Pregnancy-related costs include hospital fees, prenatal care, prenatal supplements, and birthing education.

- Nursery furniture, baby gear (such as a stroller, car seat, or cot), diapers, wipes, clothes, and feeding equipment (bottles, formula, or nursing accessories) are all necessities for families.

- Childcare: If both parents work outside the house, the cost of daycare, a nanny, or babysitting.

- Healthcare: Immunizations, out-of-pocket medical costs, pediatrician visits, and health insurance premiums.

- Education: Setting up money for books, supplies, and tuition at a university or other higher education institution.

- Extracurricular activities, toys, books, and other child-related expenditures are examples of incidental costs.

3. Establish a Parenthood Budget

Construct a thorough financial plan that takes your family's income, outlays, and savings objectives into consideration. Set aside money for both discretionary and necessary costs, including rent, utilities, food, transportation, and medical care.

- Set financial objectives and make appropriate resource allocations. A percentage of your salary should be set away for retirement contributions, emergency savings, and college funds for your offspring.
- Make adjustments to your budget to account for the additional expenditures and financial responsibilities that come with becoming a parent, such as the cost of daycare, diaper supplies, and medical bills.

4. Examine Programs for Financial Assistance

- Look into the resources and financial help programs that are available to families with children. These might include government assistance programs like Medicaid, Childcare Subsidies, WIC (Women, Infants, and Children), and SNAP (Supplemental Nutrition Assistance Program).

- Examine employer-sponsored parental leave policies such as: Employee Assistance Programs (EAPs), Flexible Spending Accounts (FSAs), Dependent Care Assistance Programs (DCAPs), and other programs that help working parents.

5. Plan for Major Life Events and Milestones

Take into account significant life events and milestones, like buying a house, upgrading to a bigger car, or making plans for your child's schooling, that might influence your family's finances. Establish deadlines and savings targets to accomplish these tasks while preserving your financial security.

- Examine your insurance policies to make sure you have enough protection for your family's financial stability, including health, life, disability, and renters or homeowners insurance.

6. Keep an Eye on and Tweak Your Financial Plan

- Review and evaluate your financial plan regularly to see how you're doing, pinpoint areas for improvement, and make any required revisions. As your family's requirements and circumstances change, update your budget accordingly. You should also occasionally review your financial objectives to make sure they're still relevant and attainable.
- Keep up with changes in tax legislation, the state of the economy, and financial trends that might affect your financial circumstances

and planning choices. See a planner or financial adviser for individualized advice and assistance based on your family's objectives and goals.

7. Adopt Smart Spending and Cheap Living Practices

To stretch your money and increase your savings, embrace smart spending and cheap living practices. Seek for ways to save costs on regular expenditures, such as buying baby supplies at a discount, utilizing rebates or coupon codes, and researching costs before making big purchases.

- To save money on daycare while maintaining high-quality care for your kid, think about other childcare options like cooperative childcare groups or nanny sharing.
- Arrange and rank family-friendly, budget-friendly activities that are both pleasant and

meaningful. Seek low-cost or free entertainment alternatives, such as public parks, neighborhood gatherings, and cultural sites.

8. Cultivate Open Communication and Financial Transparency

Discuss your family's financial objectives, values, and goals with your husband or partner. Encourage open communication and financial transparency. To guarantee agreement and support amongst parties, work together on budgetary choices, savings plans, and long-term financial planning.

- Engage older kids in talks about budgeting, money management, and responsible spending practices that are suitable for their age. Instill in them sound financial habits and abilities that will benefit them for the rest of their life.

Chapter 4

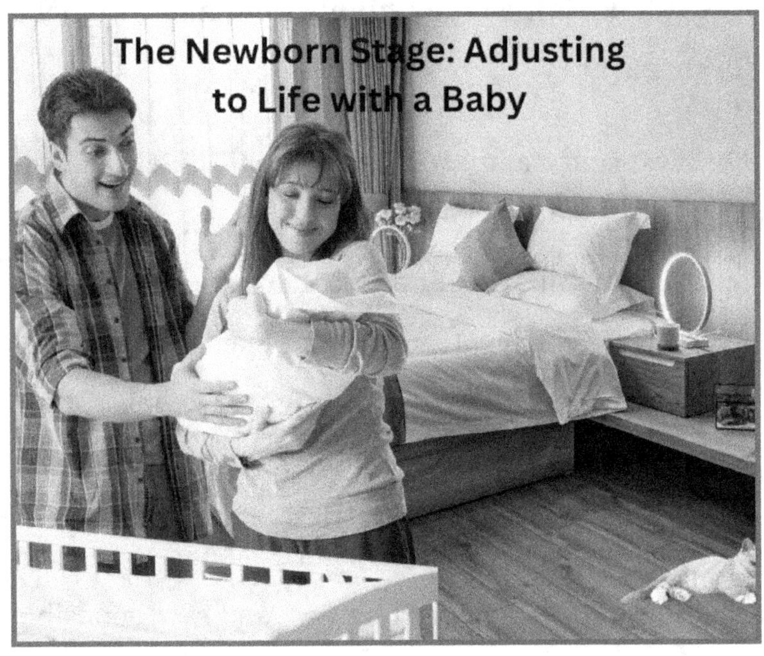

The Newborn Stage: Adjusting to Life with a Baby

A significant amount of change and adjustment occurs during the newborn stage as you welcome your child into your family and get used to your new position as parents. Here's a quick rundown of what to anticipate and how to handle this time of transition:

Physical and Emotional Changes: As you heal from delivery and get used to the responsibilities of taking care of a baby, be prepared for both physical and emotional changes. When adjusting to sleep loss, hormonal changes, and the physical demands of nursing or bottle-feeding, have patience with both yourself and your spouse.

Creating Routines: To provide yourself and your child structure and predictability, make adaptable timetables and routines. Prioritize taking care of your infant's essential requirements, such as eating, sleeping, and changing diapers, but also give yourself room to maneuver and adapt as necessary.

Seeking Support: As you negotiate the difficulties of the newborn period, don't be afraid to ask for help from friends, family, and medical experts. During this time of change, rely on your support system for comfort, emotional support, and practical help.

Bonding with Your Infant: Spend time forming a close relationship with your infant by making eye contact, touching their skin, and providing responsive care. To build a solid attachment relationship and encourage emotional connection, use tender touch, calming sounds, and caring actions.

Self-Care: As you become used to life with a baby, give your health and well-being priority. Allocate time for relaxation, and self-care pursuits that enhance your physical, emotional, and mental well-being and restore your vitality.

Managing Expectations: As you become a parent, change your priorities and expectations. Acknowledge that the infant stage is a transitory period marked by rapid modifications and adaptations, and concentrate on one day at a time.

As a couple, be in constant contact and establish a strong bond as you work through the pleasures and difficulties of parenting together. To improve your connection and relationship as a pair, schedule time for deep talks, shared experiences, and private times.

Developing a Bond with Your Infant

One of the strongest and most fulfilling bonds in life is that between a parent and their infant. Developing a close bond with your child establishes the groundwork for their future social growth, emotional health, and development. Here's a detailed look at developing a relationship with your baby:

1. Touch of Skin to Skin: Kangaroo care, or skin-to-skin contact, is an effective technique to strengthen your relationship with your infant and support their physical and mental well-being. Feel your baby's warmth, heartbeat, and aroma as you hold them to your naked chest. Skin-to-skin contact stimulates the production of hormones that promote bonding, such as oxytocin, and controls your baby's respiration, heart rate, and body temperature.

Immediately after delivery and throughout the postpartum period, establish skin-to-skin contact to enhance your relationship and encourage successful breastfeeding. Fathers and mothers may benefit from skin-to-skin contact since it gives them the chance to bond emotionally and intimately with their children.

2. Responding to Care: To foster a sense of security and trust, swiftly and sensitively respond to your baby's indications and wants. Warmth, comfort, and love are the best ways to respond to your baby's hunger signals, diaper requirements, and comfort-seeking behaviors.

When your baby cries, soothe them with soothing sounds, soft rocking, and rhythmic motions. By regularly attending to your baby's cues, you may establish a strong attachment relationship by making them feel valued, protected, and understood.

3. Maintaining Eye Contact and Effective Communication: Make eye contact with your infant to encourage communication and emotional bonding during feedings, diaper changes, and playtime. Babies react to visual signals like eye contact, gestures, and facial expressions because they are inherently attracted to faces. Use calming, melodious voices while conversing, singing, and cooing to your infant to capture their interest and promote language development. To promote reciprocal communication and social contact, tell your infant about your everyday activities, recount your exchanges, and react to their vocalizations.

4. Wearing a Baby: Keep your baby close to your body by using wraps, slings, or baby carriers throughout the day. By encouraging physical proximity, bonding, and attachment, carrying a baby helps your child feel safe and attached while you go about your everyday business.

Use a range of postures while carrying your infant to stimulate their senses, foster social contact, and foster bonding, such as hip, cradle, and upright positions. By encouraging vestibular stimulation, bodily awareness, and control, babywearing promotes child development and strengthens the link between parents and caregivers.

5. Giving and Receiving: Whether you choose to bottle feed or breastfeed, feeding time is a great chance for intimacy and connection with your child. During feeding sessions, keep your baby close to you, make eye contact, and pay attention to their indications and signals. Breastfeeding creates a special link between mother and child because it allows for skin-to-skin contact, physical intimacy, and the production of hormones that tie people together, including oxytocin.

If you're bottle-feeding, hold your baby in your arms, give them the bottle with love and gentleness, and take advantage of the chance to stare into each other's eyes and bond at feeding time. Breastfeeding is a wonderful way to nurture, soothe, and connect with your kid.

6. Light Hands and Light Massage: To help you relax, feel comfortable, and strengthen your relationship with your infant, include soft touch and massage into your everyday routine. When massaging your baby's skin, use baby-safe oils or lotions and concentrate on applying light pressure and rhythmic motions.

To encourage circulation, digestion, and relaxation, gently apply pressure and use calming strokes to massage your baby's arms, legs, back, and stomach. Observe your baby's preferences and indications, and modify your touch and pressure appropriately.

7. Play and Conversation: To strengthen your relationship with your infant and encourage their growth, engage in interactive play and sensory exercises. Engage your baby's senses and promote exploration by providing them with toys, rattles, and soft books that are age-appropriate.

During playing, spend time conversing, singing, and maintaining eye contact with your child. Encourage social engagement, communication, and connection by playing easy games like peek-a-boo, singing along to nursery songs, and gently tickling.

8. Establishing Customs and Traditions: Create regular routines and traditions that help you and your baby bond and feel connected. Establish unique times for feeding, snuggling, going to bed, and doing things together that will deepen your relationship and leave lasting memories.

To enhance your baby's feeling of identity, belonging, and cultural heritage, include family customs, cultural practices, and traditions into your everyday routine. Tell tales, sing songs, and celebrate customs that honor the history, values, and beliefs of your family.

9. Recognizing Infant Cues: Your infant uses cues and signs to express their wants and moods, so pay special attention to them. These indicators might be gestures, noises, body language, or facial expressions. Understanding your baby's cues will help you respond to them with compassion and tact, which will strengthen your relationship and establish trust.

Common cues to watch out for include crying, grimacing, making eye contact, sucking on fists or fingers, rooting (turning their head toward your touch when their cheek is stroked), and making eye contact. Because every baby is different, spend some time getting to know yours and observing their particular indications and preferences.

10. Encouraging Bonding Through Shared Sleeping: Sharing a bed with your infant, often known as co-sleeping, may strengthen your relationship with them. Frequent nocturnal feedings, soothing touch, and attentive caring are all made possible by sleeping near your infant and promoting bonding and attachment. When you practice safe co-sleeping, make sure your sleeping environment supports safe sleep habits. To lower the danger of suffocation or SIDS (Sudden Infant Death Syndrome), use a hard mattress, stay away from soft bedding and cushions, and make sure there is safe space around your infant.

11. Promoting Skin-to-Skin Contact Past the Stage of Infants: As your baby develops, skin-to-skin contact may continue to foster connection and bonding, which is advantageous even beyond the newborn period. Even as your baby becomes more autonomous and active, make skin-to-skin contact a regular part of your daily routine.

This is because skin-to-skin contact may be particularly helpful during stressful times, sickness, or developmental changes. It gives your infant emotional support, comfort, and assurance, making them feel safe and secure during trying times.

12. Developing Responsive Parenting to Build Trust: Providing for your baby's needs in a timely and considerate manner promotes trust and a stable attachment relationship. This is known as responsive parenting. Over time, your relationship with your baby will become stronger when you respond consistently to their signs and signals.

Practice responsive caring by holding, calming, and consoling your baby when they scream or show discomfort. Your kid will learn that their needs will be addressed and that they can depend on you for support and comfort if you respond to them with warmth and understanding.

13. Creating a Partner Bond with Your Newborn: It takes two parents or other caretakers to bond with their infant. Engage in joint activities like infant massage, skin-to-skin contact, and interactive play to encourage bonding and attachment as a family. Assist your spouse with caregiving duties like feeding, changing diapers, and calming your baby. Establish chances for quality time spent together and divide up the chores to strengthen your bond with your child.

14. Looking for Assistance and Resources: If you're having trouble bonding with your infant, don't be afraid to ask for help and advice from medical experts, parenting organizations, and online forums. As a parent, you're certain to encounter difficulties and failures, but there are tools available to assist you.

Enroll in parenting courses, support groups, or seminars to meet other parents, exchange stories, and gain insight from each other's triumphs and failures. Be in the company of experts, friends, and family who will support you and provide guidance, and help when required.

Essentials of Newborn Care

A baby brings pleasure and excitement to the family, but it also carries a great deal of responsibilities. Parents must be ready with the information and materials needed to meet their infant's requirements. Here is a thorough guide to the necessities of infant care:

1. Diapers

Stock up on newborn-sized disposable or cloth diapers. Newborns usually go through eight to twelve diapers in a day.

Wipes: For delicate newborn skin, use mild, hypoallergenic wipes.

Diaper Lotion: To relieve and shield your baby's skin from discomfort, have diaper rash lotion on hand.

2. Outfits and Sheets

Onesies/Bodysuits: Get a range of onesies for daytime and evening wear in newborn sizes.

Sleepers: Before going to bed, have a couple of pairs of pajamas or sleepers on.

Blankets/Swaddles: Sleep sacks or swaddling blankets may calm your infant and encourage deeper slumber.

cap and Socks: A cozy knit cap and socks will keep your newborn toasty warm.

3. Provisioning Materials

Breastfeeding: Invest in a cozy nursing bra, nursing pads, and nipple cream if you want to nurse your child.

Bottles and Formula: Prepare a few bottles, nipples, and formula (if necessary) if you want to bottle-feed your child.

Burp Cloths: To wipe up spit-up during feeding sessions, have enough supply of burp cloths on hand.

4. Cleaning and Bathing

Baby Bathtub: To bathe your baby, utilize a sink or a little bathtub designed for babies.

Baby Shampoo and Soap: For your baby's sensitive skin and hair, use mild, tear-free baby shampoo and soap.

Soft Washcloths: Keep baby-safe, soft washcloths on hand for cleaning and bathing.

Baby Brush and Comb: Gently brush and comb your baby's hair using a brush and comb with soft bristles.

5. Essentials for a Nursery

Crib or bassinet: Give your infant a secure and cozy sleeping space with a crib or bassinet.

Fitted Sheets: To avoid bunching or slippage, choose fitted crib sheets that slide over the mattress snugly.

Changing Table: Prepare a changing pad or changing table with the necessary items for changing diapers.

6. Safety and Health

Baby Thermometer: Keep an eye on your child's temperature with this digital thermometer.

Nasal Aspirator: If your infant has congestion, use a nasal aspirator or bulb syringe to empty their nasal passages.

Baby Nail Clippers: To avoid scratches, cut your baby's nails using baby-safe nail clippers or scissors.

7. Coziness and Calm

Pacifiers: Keep a couple of pacifiers around to help your infant relax in between meals.

Comfort Items: For security and comfort, provide plush animals or cozy blankets.

White Noise Machine: To help your infant sleep well, use a white noise machine or app.

8. Baby Equipment

Car Seat: Select a rear-facing seat that complies with neonatal safety regulations.

Stroller: Get your infant a stroller that is lightweight and simple to use for walks and other activities.

Baby Carrier: If you want to connect with your infant and carry them hands-free, think about getting a baby carrier or wrap.

9. Resources for Parents

Books and Online Resources: Read books, articles, and online resources to learn more about parenting and infant care.

Parenting Courses: To meet other new parents and get knowledge from seasoned experts, think about enrolling in parenting courses or joining support groups.

10. Medical Supplies

First Aid Kit: Always have a basic first aid kit on hand, filled with supplies like bandages, antiseptic wipes, and painkillers for babies.

Pediatrician Information: Keep your baby's pediatrician's contact information close to hand in case of queries or emergencies.

11. Activities and Toys for Development

To encourage early growth and excite your newborn's senses, provide toys and activities that are suitable for their age. To stimulate your baby's interest and inspire exploration, choose toys with mild noises, contrasting colors, and varied textures. You can also strengthen your baby's neck and upper body muscles and improve motor development by including stomach time in your daily routine. To guarantee your baby's safety and comfort during tummy time, choose a soft, cushioned surface and keep an eye on them.

12. Essential Travel Baby Supplies

Packing basic baby goods, such as a diaper bag filled with wipes, diapers, a changing pad, spare clothes, and feeding equipment, can help you be ready for trips and travel with your infant. Pack extra supplies and consider your baby's routine to prepare for feeding and diapering requirements while traveling. Bring along a portable baby carrier or stroller for convenient mobility and comfort on the move. When traveling with your infant, think about packing travel-sized items and accessories to reduce bulk and optimize convenience.

13. Establishing a Secure Sleep Space

By adhering to safe sleep standards, you can make sure your baby's sleeping environment is secure and supportive of sound sleep. A hard, flat crib or bassinet with a tight mattress, no loose bedding, and no soft things is the best place for your baby to sleep on their back. Wearable blankets or sleep sacks may keep your baby warm and comfortable without putting them in danger of suffocating or overheating. Make sure the room is at a reasonable temperature and don't overdress your infant before bed.

14. Developing Restful Sleep Routines

To assist your infant with unwinding and making the transition to sleep, establish a regular bedtime routine. Create a peaceful, darkly lit sleeping space away from distractions like bright lights or loud sounds to promote good sleep patterns. Incorporate relaxing activities like silent snuggling, bath time, and gentle massage to indicate that it's time for sleep. Maintaining a regular sleep schedule and adhering to a predictable bedtime routine can help your baby's natural sleep-wake cycles.

Chapter 5

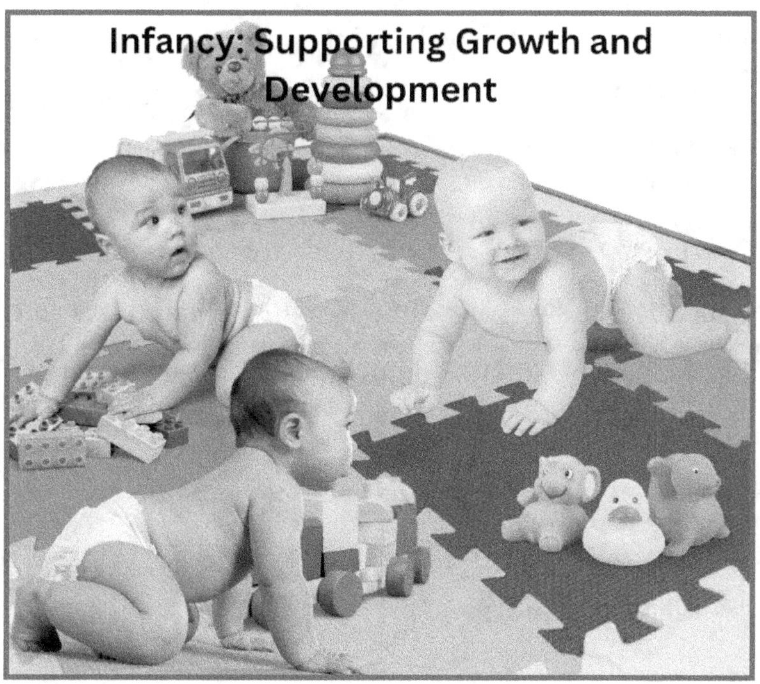

Chapter 5

Infancy: Supporting Growth and Development

It is essential to foster growth and development in early childhood to establish the groundwork for a child's success and well-being throughout life. Here is a brief guide on how to promote the growth and development of infants:

Nutrition: Make sure babies are getting enough food by nursing or using formula. Antibodies and vital nutrients included in breast milk encourage a strong immune system and healthy development. Adhere to the suggested feeding recommendations and progressively introduce solid meals as directed by medical authorities.

Providing caring and attentive care is essential to meeting the physical and emotional requirements of newborns. To foster bonding and attachment, swiftly respond to indications for food, pain, and comfort. You may also encourage pleasant interactions like snuggling, chatting, and singing.

Encourage stomach Time: To aid in the development of an infant's shoulder, back, and neck muscles, it is recommended to encourage supervised stomach time. Additionally to promoting motor development, tummy time helps avoid flat patches on the back of the skull.

Encourage Sensory Exploration: To help babies' growing senses, expose them to a range of sensory experiences. Play with water, sand, or soft materials, or participate in other activities that promote sensory exploration. Provide toys with a variety of textures, colors, noises, and forms.

Promote Motor Development: Give babies the chance to move and explore to aid in their motor development. Provide playthings and toys that are safe and developmentally appropriate to promote reaching, gripping, rolling, crawling, and ultimately walking.

Establish habits: To help newborns feel safe and develop a feeling of predictability and stability in their surroundings, establish regular habits for eating, resting, and playing. Regular schedules help babies regulate their emotions and encourage sound sleep habits.

Encourage the development of language in babies by talking to them often and reacting to their coos, babbling, and gestures. Engage in engaging activities like reading books, singing songs, and playing peek-a-boo to foster language development and communication skills. Label objects and behaviors using basic, repeated words.

To ensure that babies sleep in a safe environment, turn them onto their backs and place them on a firm mattress free of soft items or loose linen. To lower the risk of sleep-related accidents and sudden infant death syndrome (SIDS), adhere to recommended safe sleep habits.

Track Developmental Milestones: If you are concerned about an infant's growth, keep track of their developmental milestones and seek advice from medical authorities. Pediatricians recommend regular checkups to evaluate growth and development and to provide early intervention when necessary.

Give Unconditional Love and Support: To promote an infant's emotional health and feeling of security, give them unwavering love, affection, and support. Establish a loving atmosphere that fosters trust and connection by being kind and sensitive to their wants and feelings.

Let's now explore this in more detail in the subsections that follow.

Understanding Baby Milestones

The developmental accomplishments and skills that newborns gain throughout the first year of life are referred to as infant milestones. These developmental milestones include a range of areas related to your baby's physical, cognitive, social, and emotional growth and advancement. Parents and other caregivers must be aware of newborn milestones to monitor their child's growth, spot any possible issues, and provide the right kind of support and stimulation. This is a thorough examination of baby milestones in many domains:

A. Physical Development: During the first year of life, infants grow and develop physically quickly, reaching notable milestones like:

i. Gross Motor Skills: Crawling, walking, running, leaping, climbing, and balancing are examples of motions that require the use of vast muscle groups. These abilities, which come gradually throughout life, are crucial for coordination and movement. The following lists the gross motor milestones:

Infanthood (0–12 months): Infants progressively learn to regulate their muscles and movements throughout the first year of life. They start by raising their heads, rolling over, and sitting up with assistance. Eventually, they will learn to pull themselves up to stand, crawl, and glide over furniture.

Toddlerhood (ages 1-3): During this time, children develop their gross motor abilities and become more mobile on their own. They pick up the skills necessary to run, leap with both feet, kick a ball, climb stairs with help, and ride a tricycle.

Preschool Years (3-6 Years): During this time, children continue to develop their coordination and gross motor abilities. They can hop on one foot, skip, jump rope, run more steadily, climb playground equipment, and toss and catch balls with more precision.

School-Age Years (6–12 Years): Children in this age group engage in increasingly difficult physical activities and continue to refine their gross motor abilities. They participate in sports and leisure activities, hone their running, leaping, and throwing abilities, and build their strength, agility, and endurance.

ii. Fine Motor Skills: Hand-eye coordination, object manipulation, and grasping are examples of precise motions that require the utilization of tiny muscle groups. These abilities are essential for writing, sketching, cutting, and self-care duties. A summary of fine motor milestones is provided below:

Infanthood (0–12 months): Babies start to explore and handle items with their hands, grab toys, and put things in their mouths to taste them. With increased dexterity, they learn to move toys and pick up tiny things with their fingers (pincer grip).

Toddlerhood (ages 1-3): During this time, children develop their fine motor abilities and increase their hand control. They can flip pages in a book, stack blocks, feed themselves with cutlery, draw with crayons, and handle tiny items like beads and puzzle pieces.

The preschool years (ages 3-6): At this stage, children continue to hone their fine motor abilities and take part in more complex activities. They can precisely manage little things, cut with scissors along a straight line, trace letters and basic forms, and handle small objects.

School-Age Years (6–12 years): Children in this age group continue to hone their fine motor abilities and become adept at activities like typing, handwriting, creating intricate drawings, tying shoelaces, and precisely manipulating tools and utensils.

The following factors affect physical development

Children's physical development is influenced by several variables, including their surroundings, play and physical exercise opportunities, diet, and heredity. It is crucial to provide kids with plenty of chances to exercise, play outside, and explore to encourage good physical development. Promoting physical activities that test children's gross and fine motor skills like climbing, swinging, block-building, and sports, help them gain strength, coordination, and self-assurance in their physical capabilities.

Promoting the physical development of Children's physical development is greatly aided by parents and other caregivers who provide a safe, stimulating environment that promotes movement and discovery. Here are some strategies that encourage kids' physical development:

i. Give kids the chance to play and move actively both indoors and outside.

ii. Provide a selection of toys and equipment that are age-appropriate and encourage the development of both fine and gross motor abilities.

iii. Encourage your kids to participate in physical activities that build strength and coordination, such as gymnastics, dancing, and sports.

iv. Get your family moving and provide an example of a healthy, active lifestyle.

v. Make sure kids have access to wholesome meals and enough sleep to promote their general development.

B. Cognitive Development: The expansion and improvement of a child's mental abilities, such as their capacity for thought, language, learning, problem-solving, memory, and attention, is referred to as cognitive development. It includes how kids see, comprehend, and engage with the world around them in addition to their capacity for information acquisition and application. Here is a more thorough examination of children's cognitive development:

1. Stage II (from birth to two years old)

Infants increasingly gain knowledge of the environment via their perceptions and movements throughout the sensorimotor period. During this phase, important cognitive benchmarks include:

Object Permanence: Infants learn that things exist even when they are hidden from view at the age of 6 to 8 months. An infant demonstrates this milestone by reaching for a covered toy or by searching for a concealed item.

Cause and Effect: When a rattle is shaken to produce sound or a toy is pressed to activate, an infant begins to comprehend cause-and-effect connections. Through trial and error, they pick up knowledge and start to consider the effects of their actions.

Symbolic Play: As the sensorimotor period comes to a close, babies play symbolic roles. Examples of this kind of play include acting out feeding a doll or using objects to symbolize other things. This illustrates the origins of imaginative and symbolic cognition.

2. Stage Before Operation (2–7 Years)

Although toddlers start to think symbolically and acquire linguistic abilities during the preoperational period, much of their thinking is still egocentric and concrete. During this phase, important cognitive benchmarks include:

Language Development: Youngsters pick up language quickly and expand their vocabulary, which helps them communicate their needs and wants more clearly. They converse with people by asking questions, holding discussions, and using words.

Symbolic Thinking: Through role-playing, storytelling, and creative play, children exhibit symbolic thinking. They participate in pretend play and use objects to symbolize other things, exhibiting a comprehension of symbolic representation.

Egocentrism: Kids often perceive the world from their perspective and struggle to comprehend the viewpoints of others. Their egocentric mentality may cause them to struggle with sharing, taking turns, and empathy.

3. Stage of Concrete Operation (7 to 11 years)

Though their thinking is still restricted to physical, palpable experiences, toddlers become more rational and capable of comprehending abstract ideas throughout the concrete operational stage. During this phase, important cognitive benchmarks include:

Conservation: Kids learn to comprehend that even when a substance's form or arrangement changes, its volume or amount stays the same. They know, for instance, that adding water to a short, broad glass from a tall, narrow glass does not increase the volume of water in the glass.

Classification and Seriation: Kids can group items into groups according to similar qualities and put them in a sensible sequence. They can classify items based on their understanding of concepts like size, form, color, and number.

Logical Reasoning: Kids start to think more methodically and rationally, using both deductive and inductive reasoning to solve issues. They are better at precisely understanding cause-and-effect linkages and can solve problems by following a set of processes.

Encourage children to solve issues on their own and with others by teaching them how to effectively communicate, think critically, and resolve conflicts. Give them the chance to experience handling problems in authentic settings and be there to provide advice and assistance when required.

Develop Kindness and Empathy: Encourage acts of kindness and generosity, encourage perspective-taking and empathy for others, and model compassionate and caring conduct.

Teach Social Skills: Through play, group activities, and cooperative projects, provide kids the chance to practice social skills including sharing, taking turns, listening, and collaborating. Encourage and provide feedback to strengthen constructive social habits.

Establish a Positive atmosphere: Establish an atmosphere that is welcoming to all people, celebrates individual variety, and fosters justice, empathy, and respect. Teach kids to value each other's individuality and to welcome diversity.

C. The term "communication and language development": This describes how children gradually pick up and hone abilities linked to comprehending and utilizing language for social interaction, thinking and emotional expression, and knowledge of their surroundings. It includes all facets of language, such as speaking, writing, listening, and reading, and it is essential to the cognitive, social, and emotional growth of an individual. Here's a more thorough look at how children's language and communication develop:

1. Prelinguistic Communication (0 - 12 Months)

Infants communicate nonverbally during the prelinguistic period by using gestures, facial expressions, and vocalizations. Important turning points in this phase include:

Cooing and Babbling: As they explore with vocalizations, infants start to generate vowel sounds (like "cooing") and consonant-vowel combinations (like "babbling").

Joint Attention: Babies learn to follow a caregiver's gaze or point at interesting items to share their attention with others.

Turn-Taking: Babies participate in early dialogues with their caretakers, voicing their opinions and offering their responses in turn.

2. Initial Language Acquisition (12 to 24 Months)

Toddlers start to form words throughout the early stages of language development, and they also start to increase their vocabulary. Important turning points in this phase include:

First Words: Between the ages of 12 and 18 months, toddlers usually say their first words, which are usually references to familiar places, people, or activities.

Vocabulary Expansion: Through interactions with caregivers and spoken language exposure, toddlers quickly pick up new words and start to expand their vocabulary.

Small, one- or two-word telegraphic phrases are used by toddlers to communicate their fundamental needs and wants (e.g., "more milk," "big dog").

3. Development of Grammar and Vocabulary (2 to 5 Years):

Preschoolers continue to grow in their linguistic abilities and pick up more sophisticated grammar and vocabulary at this time. Important turning points in this phase include:

Quick Vocabulary Growth: Kids go through a "vocabulary explosion," picking up new words quickly and expanding their vocabulary base to include nouns, verbs, adjectives, and other speech elements.

Sentence Structure: Kids start using questions and compound sentences, among other more complicated sentence forms.

Grammar Development: Youngsters learn the fundamentals of grammar, including word order, tense, and subject-verb agreement.

4. School-Age Years: Language Use and Comprehension:

Children continue to hone their language abilities throughout the school years and utilize language for a range of objectives, such as understanding spoken and written language, communication, and the expression of ideas and emotions. Important turning points in this phase include:

Children acquire literacy abilities and comprehension techniques for deciphering written texts as they learn to read and write.

Narrative Skills: Kids learn how to tell and comprehend tales, which includes putting events in order, character and location descriptions, and theme and major concept identification.

Conversational Skills: Children use language to discuss ideas, ask questions, express views, and negotiate meanings in interactions with peers and adults.

Elements Affecting Language and Communication Development

Children's language and communication development is influenced by several elements, including social interactions, language exposure, environment, and heredity. Language development and literacy abilities are enhanced when children are exposed to rich and engaging language experiences, such as books, discussions, spoken language, and interactions with classmates and caregivers.

fostering the development of language and communication

Through the provision of chances for meaningful interactions, exposure to rich language experiences, and explicit training in language and literacy skills, parents, caregivers, and educators play a crucial role in fostering children's language and communication development. The following are some strategies to aid with children's language and communication development:

Talk to the Kids: Talk to the kids by asking open-ended questions, encouraging them to share their ideas and experiences, and paying attention to what they have to say.

Read Aloud: Encourage youngsters to interact with books and tales by reading aloud to them regularly. Encourage kids to conclude, draw connections, and make predictions as you discuss the themes, characters, and storyline.

Provide Language-Rich Environments: Establish language-rich settings where kids may interact with books, songs, rhymes, and discussions, among other spoken and written language experiences.

Extend children's remarks, utilize descriptive language, introduce new vocabulary terms in context, and provide an example of rich and diverse language usage.

Promote Storytelling and Creative Expression: Inspire kids to use their imaginations for role-playing, storytelling, and creative expression via writing, drawing, and role-playing.

Encourage Literacy abilities: Through exercises like reading, writing, and word games, provide kids the chance to polish literacy abilities including phonemic awareness, letter identification, and comprehension techniques.

Encouraging Restful Sleep Practices

Encouraging children to sleep properly is crucial for their mental, emotional, and physical health. Getting enough sleep promotes healthy growth and development, improves memory consolidation and learning, controls mood and behavior, and fortifies the immune system. This is a thorough tutorial on helping kids develop good sleeping habits:

1. Create a Regular Bedtime Schedule: Establish a soothing bedtime routine that lets your kids know when it's time to unwind and get ready for bed. To help your kids' internal clocks work, try starting the routine at the same time every night.

2. Establish a Calm Sleep Environment: Reduce light, noise, and distractions in the sleeping area to promote peaceful sleep. Make sure your bedding is comfy and your room is kept at a suitable temperature (preferably between 65 and 70°F or 18 and 21°C).

3. Limit your screen time before night: Set aside time before bed for your kid to use screens to help their brain relax and get ready for sleep. Try to avoid exposing them to displays as stimulating as TVs, laptops, cellphones, and tablets at least an hour before bed.

4. Promote Movement Throughout the Day: Avoid doing intense exercise just before bedtime as it may invigorate your kid and make it more difficult for them to fall asleep. Instead, encourage your child to play outside and engage in regular physical activity throughout the day to encourage peaceful sleep at night.

5. Track Your Sugar and Caffeine Intake: Restrict your child's intake of caffeine and sugary meals and beverages, particularly in the hours before bed. These substances may interfere with sleep and disturb the body's normal circadian rhythm.

6. Clarify Your Sleep Expectations: Together with your kid, set clear expectations and limits for their sleep, stressing the need for regular bedtimes and wake-up hours. Also, explain to them the significance of sleep for their general health and well-being and let them help create their bedtime routine.

7. Instruct on Relaxation Methods: To help your kid relax and wind down before bed, teach them relaxation methods like progressive muscle relaxation, deep breathing, or visualization. Then, use these techniques together throughout the evening routines to further encourage tranquility and relaxation.

8. Handle Your Anxiety and Fears at Night: To help your kid sleep better, encourage open conversation and give assistance in resolving any underlying worries or concerns. Validate your child's thoughts and fears about going to bed and offer comfort and reassurance as required.

9. Track Sleep Patterns and Make Adjustments as Required: Keep an eye on your child's sleeping habits and behaviors, and adapt their sleep schedule accordingly. Be accommodating to your child's unique sleep requirements while keeping regular bedtimes and wake-up times.

10. If Needed, Seek Professional Assistance: Seeking advice from a pediatrician or sleep specialist may be necessary if your child constantly struggles with sleep issues despite your best efforts to instill healthy sleep habits. Improving your child's overall health and quality of sleep may require addressing underlying medical conditions or sleep disorders.

Chapter *6*

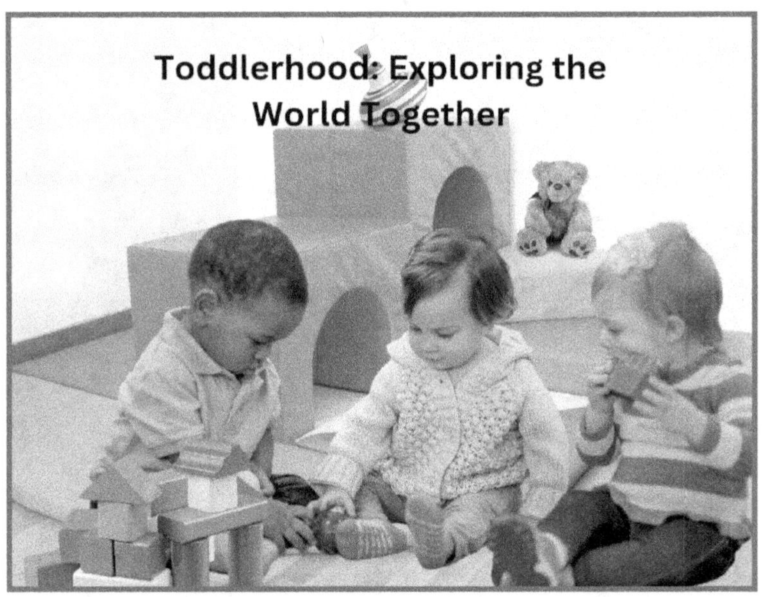

Chapter 6

Toddlerhood: Exploring the World Together

The toddler years are an amazing developmental time characterized by fast growth, curiosity, and discovery. As toddlers go from infancy to early childhood, they experience significant changes. A growing sense of curiosity and an unwavering desire to learn more about the world around them define this time.

Toddlers are curious learners who avidly take in knowledge from everything they touch, taste, smell, see, and hear. They are like little scientists. Learning may be gained from every experience, whether it is playing in the puddles, building with blocks, or examining insects in the garden.

Toddlers enthusiastically explore limits and strive for autonomy in their activities as they start to establish their individuality. Even seemingly little activities like dressing, feeding oneself, and toy selection become significant chances for mastery and self-expression. During this phase, parents are crucial because they provide toddlers with direction and encouragement while giving them the flexibility to explore and learn at their speed.

A child's language develops quickly throughout the toddler years when they start learning new words and putting them together to make phrases. Toddlers may still have a little vocabulary, but communication becomes a strong instrument for them to convey their needs, wants, and feelings. By having talks with their children, reading aloud to them, and identifying things and activities in their surroundings, parents may encourage language development in their children.

Another characteristic of toddlerhood is social-emotional development, as kids learn how to manage their emotions and interact with others.

Toddlers may feel a broad variety of emotions as they adjust to their newfound independence and the difficulties of sharing and taking turns, from happiness and enthusiasm to frustration and wrath. By modeling empathy, teaching conflict resolution techniques, and creating plenty of opportunities for healthy social interactions with classmates and family, parents may support their toddlers' social skill development.

Promoting Language Acquisition

It is crucial to support children's language development to promote social connection, cognitive growth, and communication abilities. Check out these brief manuals for promoting children's language development:

Talk to Your Kid: Throughout the day, have meaningful and regular talks with your kid. Discuss your activities, your child's activities, and the things you see in your environment. To aid with vocabulary reinforcement, speak simply and use essential terms several times.

Read Aloud: Starting at a young age, read to your kid regularly. Pick a range of books with repeating phrases, rhymes, and vibrant illustrations. Asking questions, pointing to visuals, and making predictions about what will happen next can all help to get your youngster involved.

Sing Songs and Nursery Rhymes: Children learn rhythm and phonological awareness via singing songs and nursery rhymes. Select upbeat, engaging music with memorable melodies that promote involvement and repeat listening.

When your kid talks, give them more space to express themselves in words and sentences. This will help them learn new vocabulary and provide proper grammar. When your toddler says "car," for instance, you may answer, "Yes, that's a big black car."

Encourage Pretend Play: Using their imaginations and using language in context, youngsters may benefit from pretend play. Give your kids props and let them pretend to be in other roles, like a doctor, a grocery shop, or a home.

Give Your Youngster the Chance to Interact Socially: Encourage your youngster to engage in social interactions with peers and adults. Children may practice communication skills, take turns, and learn from others via playdates, preschool, and community events.

Use Body Language and Gestures: To enhance verbal communication, use body language, gestures, and facial expressions. Reinforce meaning and aid comprehension by pointing to items, making eye contact, and using hand gestures.

Be Kind and Patient: Give your youngster time to comprehend and react to language. Refrain from overcorrecting or pressing your kid; instead, be kind and gentle with them. Along the process, acknowledge their accomplishments and encourage them.

By putting these techniques into practice, parents and other adults may provide a nurturing atmosphere for language development and assist kids in developing lifelong communication skills.

Positive Toddler Discipline Methods

Toddlers might benefit from positive disciplinary methods that emphasize building a strong bond between parents and children while educating and guiding conduct courteously and compassionately. Without resorting to force or punishment, these strategies seek to establish clear boundaries, impart valuable life skills, and promote positive behaviors.

A detailed summary of toddler-friendly positive discipline methods is provided below:

Set Age-appropriate and Definable Expectations: Clearly define the conduct you anticipate from your child. In plain words, express your expectations clearly, and make sure you repeat them often. Rather than telling someone to "don't run," you may tell them to "walk slowly indoors."

Be a Positive Role Model: Since kids pick up behavior from their parents, set a good example for them. Show your youngster how to behave and think by modeling virtues like patience, compassion, and respect for others. Since your behavior speaks louder than words, make an effort to live up to the morals you want your kid to learn.

Employ good Reinforcement: Provide incentives, encouragement, and praise to reinforce good behavior. Recognize and praise your child when they demonstrate positive actions, like sharing with a friend or handling a pet gently. To emphasize what they accomplished, give them particular appreciation. For example, "I like how you shared your toy with your friend." "You were extremely sweet to say that."

Redirect Negative Behavior: Draw your toddler's attention to things that are more suitable rather than what they should not be doing. Provide substitute options or diversions to assist them in diverting their attention from unwanted acts. If your child is tossing toys, for instance, gently divert their focus to a new game or object.

Communicate with your youngster using positive words, emphasizing their abilities rather than their limitations. Consider stating, "Let's walk together," as an alternative to, "No running." To help your child behave appropriately and encourage good decisions, speak to them in an upbeat and supportive manner.

Set Boundaries and Limitations: To assist your child in understanding what is expected of them, set boundaries and limitations that are consistent and unambiguous. Be calm and strong in communicating expectations and standards, and make sure they are constantly enforced.

When necessary, be ready to provide helpful reminders and direction; but, refrain from using coercion or threats of harm to compel compliance.

Promote Problem-Solving: Motivate your young child to solve problems and come up with answers to disputes or difficulties. Give your kids the freedom to come up with their answers for handling problems or getting over difficulties rather than forcing them to adopt yours. As required, provide assistance and direction, but let your child participate actively in problem-solving.

Use Time-In Rather Than Time-Out: To assist your baby learn to control their emotions and settle down, try using time-ins as an alternative to punishing strategies like time-outs. In times of difficulty, provide your kid with consolation and encouragement, and assist them in recognizing and expressing their emotions healthily. Instead of using these times to penalize people, use them as teaching and connecting opportunities.

Be Kind and Patient: Toddlers are still learning and growing, so show them kindness and patience as they deal with the transition to adulthood. Offer support and confidence when things become tough, and demonstrate empathy and compassion for their feelings and challenges. Reassure them that it's OK for them to feel angry or annoyed by validating their emotions.

Retain Consistency: Positive discipline relies heavily on consistency. Maintain consistency in your standards, guidelines, and sanctions, and honor your word. Predictability and regularity are what children love, so being consistent will help your toddler feel safe and know what's expected of them.

Getting Ready for School

A child's preparation for preschool is an exciting turning point in their educational path, one that both parents and children should celebrate. Preparing for preschool comprises several important actions to guarantee a seamless transition and provide the ideal environment for learning. This is a thorough rundown on how to be ready for preschool:

Investigate Preschool Alternatives: To pick a program that fits your child's requirements, interests, and family values, start by investigating the many preschool alternatives available in your community.

Think about things like schedule, location, curriculum, instructor credentials, and learning style. See prospective preschools in person, ask questions, and take note of events in the classroom to have a feel for the setting and pedagogy.

Create a pattern: It may be difficult for young children to adjust to a preschool schedule, so it's beneficial to create a reliable daily pattern at home. Establish consistent wake-up, dinner, and sleep schedules to aid your youngster in acclimating to a regimented routine. Engage in self-help activities like dressing, using the restroom, and hand washing to encourage self-sufficiency and get your kid ready for preschool responsibilities.

Encourage Social Skills: It's important to assist your kid in developing social skills before entering school since preschool offers priceless opportunities for social engagement and peer interactions. Set up playdates with classmates, take your kids to parks or community centers, and sign them up for group activities like painting or music lessons to promote sociability and teamwork.

Practice Separation: Before your child's first day of preschool, it's crucial to gradually introduce separation if they haven't spent much time apart from you. Start with shorter separations; for example, leave your kid for short amounts of time with a family member or trusted caretaker. To assist your kid get used to being away from you, gradually lengthen the time that they spend apart from you.

Promote Independence: Self-help abilities and independence should be fostered in preschoolers at home since they will be expected to take on more responsibilities and duties on their own. Help your kid learn how to put on clothes, load their bag, and follow basic directions without your continual monitoring. Let your kid make decisions and assume age-appropriate tasks to foster problem-solving and decision-making abilities.

Practice School Readiness Skills: It's beneficial to have preschoolers practice school readiness skills at home as they are exposed to a range of academic ideas and abilities. Through exercises like reading books, singing songs, counting items, and investigating letters and numbers, put your attention on fostering early literacy and numeracy abilities. Embrace exploratory play and hands-on activities to foster curiosity and a passion for learning.

Include Your Kid in the Planning Process: Create a transition plan to assist your kid in acclimating to the new schedule and surroundings of preschool.

Changes to your child's daily routine, such as getting up earlier and practicing being alone for brief periods, should be gradually included. Allowing your kid to choose a lunchbox, bag, and other supplies is another way to include them. Let them choose a special dress for their first day and help fill their rucksack with necessities like a water bottle, a snack, and a change of clothes. Your kid will feel more enthusiastic and involved in their preschool experience if you include them in the planning process.

Encourage Emotional Resilience: Before the first day of school, it's important to encourage emotional resilience and confidence in children, since the start of preschool may be an emotional time for them.

Have a good, comforting conversation with your kid about preschool, focusing on the wonderful and exciting things they will experience. Throughout the transition process, give your kid plenty of emotional support and confidence while also validating their emotions and anxieties.

Visit the Preschool: Before your child's first day, take them on a tour of the preschool to acquaint them with the setting and introduce them to their instructor. Together, spend time visiting the classroom, playground, and other school grounds. If at all feasible, introduce your kid to their instructor and other students. Preschool visits may ease your child's transition and reduce feelings of worry and uncertainty.

Speaking with the Preschool Staff: Maintain open lines of contact with the preschool staff to discuss your child's abilities, interests, and any worries you may have. Give pertinent information about your child's habits, preferences, and any necessary special accommodations.

Work together with the preschool to create plans for assisting your child's transition and resolving any issues that may come up.

Finally, commemorate this significant turning point in your child's life by praising their accomplishments and recognizing their development. Make the first day of preschool a happy and memorable occasion for your kid by taking pictures, crafting a unique memento, or organizing a little party.

Chapter 7

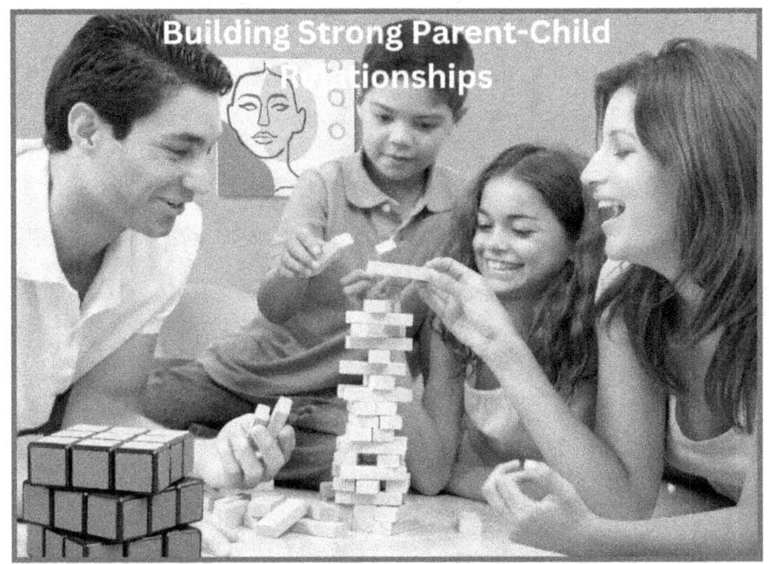

Chapter 7

Building Strong Parent-Child Relationships

To support healthy growth, emotional well-being, and good communication and connection between parents and children, strong parent-child ties must be built. The following are essential tactics and methods for developing wholesome parent-child relationships:

Unconditional Love and Acceptance: Regardless of your child's actions or achievements, show them your undying love and acceptance. Tell them that you appreciate and admire them for who they are, not simply for what they do.

Active Listening: When speaking with your kid, engage in active listening. Maintain eye contact, give them your whole attention, and seem as if you want to hear what they have to say. Don't interrupt or minimize their ideas and views; instead, validate their experiences and emotions, and also Promote polite and honest conversation.

Empathy and Understanding: Be empathetic and understanding of the feelings and experiences of your kid. Consider yourself in their position and acknowledge their emotions, even if you don't always share them. Encourage them by being there for them in trying times and by celebrating their victories and happiness.

Maintaining consistency and predictability is important when interacting with your kid. Create routines and limits that provide people with a feeling of security and consistency, and be sure to regularly implement penalties and incentives. This fosters a sense of safety and security in your child's bond with you.

Respect and Trust: Show your kid that you believe in their skills and judgment while also treating them with decency and respect. When it is appropriate, include children in decision-making processes. At the same time, give them the freedom to assume age-appropriate responsibilities and make their own decisions.

Good Discipline: Apply constructive, positive discipline that prioritizes guidance and instruction above punishment. Establish limits and expectations that are clear, then apply them with compassion and understanding. Make the most of your child's punishment to teach them from their errors and help them make better decisions in the future.

Physical Affection: Give your kid hugs, kisses, and cuddles to show them how much you care. Physical contact strengthens the emotional connection between a parent and their kid and is a potent means of expressing love and affection.

Good Family Time: Make time each day for your family to gather together and strengthen your bonds as a unit. This might include common interests and hobbies, game evenings, lunches, and trips with the family.

Individual Attention: To foster individual interactions and strengthen your bond with your children, try to set aside time each day for one-on-one time. This might include customized activities, chats, or special trips based on the needs and interests of each kid.

Flexibility and Adaptability: Recognize that every kid is different and may need various approaches and supports. Be flexible and adaptive in your parenting style. Be prepared to modify your parenting approach in response to your child's shifting requirements, temperament, and developmental stage.

Strengthening Family Ties Through Shared Activities

One of the most effective ways to build a feeling of togetherness and belonging among family members, create enduring memories, and strengthen family relationships is via shared activities. Engaging in shared activities offers chances for meaningful engagement, enjoyable times, and quality time spent together.

Here's a thorough examination of how family relationships may be reinforced via shared activities:

Making Memorable Experiences: Engaging in shared activities helps families to construct priceless memories that will last a lifetime. Whether it's a simple game night at home, a Christmas ritual, or a family trip, these shared experiences contribute to the history of the family and strengthen the bonds that bind them together.

Encouraging Open Communication and Deeper Connections: Engaging in shared activities helps to promote open communication and stronger bonds among family members. Having fun and interacting with others creates a natural setting for connecting, laughing, and talking. Engaging in activities together gives family members a comfortable and encouraging space to talk about their ideas, emotions, and experiences.

Establishing Trust and Support: Engaging in shared activities as a family enhances the support network inside the family. Family members learn to trust and rely on one another by spending quality time together and participating in fulfilling activities. This support network bolsters the idea that family members can always rely on one another and acts as a safety net during trying times.

Fostering collaboration and Teamwork: A lot of shared activities call for collaboration and teamwork, which may strengthen links within the family and encourage a feeling of oneness. Engaging in cooperative activities like solving puzzles together, playing team sports, or working together on family projects fosters effective communication, problem-solving skills, and a sense of accomplishment when accomplishments are reached collectively.

Managing Conflict: Parents should instill in their children healthy means of resolving disputes and conflicts since conflict is an inevitable aspect of sibling relationships. Siblings should be encouraged to resolve conflicts amicably by taking turns, making concessions, and coming up with win-win solutions. Instruct them on how to politely and assertively communicate their emotions, and provide direction and encouragement as they resolve disputes together. As you engage with siblings, provide an example of good conflict resolution techniques and assist them in identifying when they need adult assistance to settle disputes.

Encouraging Individuality and Autonomy: Honor and cherish the distinctive qualities, hobbies, and personalities of each sibling, and support them in pursuing their interests and objectives. Sibling rivalry and favoritism should be avoided since they might lead to animosity and rivalry within the family. Create chances for siblings to share their accomplishments and abilities, and encourage them to appreciate and support each other's victories.

Encouraging Emotional Well-Being: By lowering stress, encouraging relaxation, and cultivating happy feelings, engaging in activities together may benefit family members' emotional well-being. Laughter, pleasure, and enjoyment are produced when family members participate in rewarding and pleasurable activities together. This may reduce stress and reinforce emotional links.

Teaching Values and Life Lessons: Parents may impart valuable life lessons and values to their children via shared activities. Participating in sports may teach children the value of collaboration, sportsmanship, and persistence. Similarly, engaging in creative efforts can help children develop their creativity and problem-solving abilities. In the framework of the family, shared activities provide invaluable chances for learning and development.

Encouraging Healthy Development: Taking part in family-friendly activities promotes healthy growth through life. Engaging in joint activities with parents and siblings helps children grow socially, emotionally, and cognitively. It also helps them feel safe and included. Adults may find satisfaction outside of work and other duties, de-stress, and reestablish relationships with loved ones via shared hobbies.

Managing Personal Time and Parenting Responsibilities

Maintaining a healthy and meaningful lifestyle as a parent requires striking a balance between parental obligations and personal leisure. Prioritizing their interests, well-being, and self-care is just as vital for parents as prioritizing their children's needs.

Parents may prevent burnout, lessen stress, and promote more satisfaction and fulfillment in both their family life and personal endeavors by striking the correct balance between parenting and personal leisure. Here's a thorough examination of methods for striking this balance:

Make Self-Care a Priority: Understand that looking after your needs is not selfish but rather necessary for your general well-being and capacity to be a good parent. Prioritize your well-being by setting aside time each day to partake in rejuvenating and recharging activities. Exercise, mindfulness, reading, hobbies, and quality time with friends and family are a few examples of this. You'll be more capable of managing the responsibilities of parenting and overcoming obstacles with more resilience and optimism if you put self-care first.

Establish Limits: To guarantee that you have time set aside for yourself, clearly define the limits between your time and your parenting duties. Share these limits with your family and create expectations and routines that help you meet your desire for alone time. Set firm limits and refrain from taking on too many commitments or activities that interfere with your time.

Nourish Your Body: Give your physical health priority by feeding it a balanced diet, getting regular exercise, and getting enough sleep. Eat meals that are high in nutrients and provide your body the energy and vigor it needs. Schedule regular exercise to help you feel better mentally, and physically, and minimize stress. Make sleep a priority and create a regular sleep schedule that enables you to have enough restorative sleep every night. Maintaining your physical health sets the stage for your general health and vigor.

Take Part in the Things You Love: Schedule time for the things that make you happy, fulfilled, and purposeful. Make time for the things that feed your spirit and stoke your enthusiasm a priority, whether it's engaging in a new interest, taking up a pastime, or spending time with loved ones. Taking part in the things you enjoy may lower stress, improve mood, and improve general well-being.

Practice Self-Compassion: Show yourself kindness and compassion, particularly when you're going through a tough period. Be kind, sympathetic, and empathic to yourself as you would imagine a friend going through a similar ordeal. Recognize your humanity, accept your flaws, and embrace yourself with unwavering love and acceptance to cultivate self-compassion. Remind yourself that, just as you are, you are deserving of compassion, love, and care.

Arrange and Schedule: Be proactive in your time management by arranging and organizing your activities as well as your parental duties. To schedule time for significant family responsibilities, such as extracurricular activities, school functions, and housework, utilize a planner or calendar. Whether you set aside time for self-care and relaxation on a daily, weekly, or monthly basis, make sure you schedule personal time for yourself and consider it as an absolute need.

Assign and Divide Obligations: To relieve yourself of some of the burdens of parenthood, don't be scared to assign duties and obligations to other family members or caretakers. If applicable, split up the childcare obligations with your spouse, and include older kids in age-appropriate home tasks and responsibilities. When you need time to unwind and concentrate on your interests and needs, enlist the assistance of friends, extended family, or babysitters.

Practice Time Management: To maximize your available time and save wasted time, use efficient time management techniques. To increase productivity, rank jobs according to their significance and urgency and then methodically approach them. Seek ways to automate tedious jobs, simplify routines, and cut out time-consuming pursuits that take away from your time.

Set Reasonable Expectations: As a parent, try not to place unreasonably high standards on yourself and accept that you won't always be flawless. Give yourself permission to put your own needs first, to follow your hobbies and passions, and to do so guilt-free. Recognize that there will be moments when taking care of your children comes before personal time, but make an effort to strike a balance that enables you to fulfill your needs as a person and your parental obligations.

Communicate Openly: Be honest and transparent with your family about the value of self-care and your need for personal time. Encourage your spouse, kids, and other family members to share their thoughts, worries, and limits with you. By creating an environment that values candid communication and mutual assistance, you may collaborate to discover solutions that strike a balance between everyone's needs and objectives.

Be Adaptive and Flexible: Realize that striking a balance between personal time and parental obligations is a continuous process that may call for modifications and adaptations over time. When your family's demands change, be prepared to modify your routines and priorities.

Chapter *8*

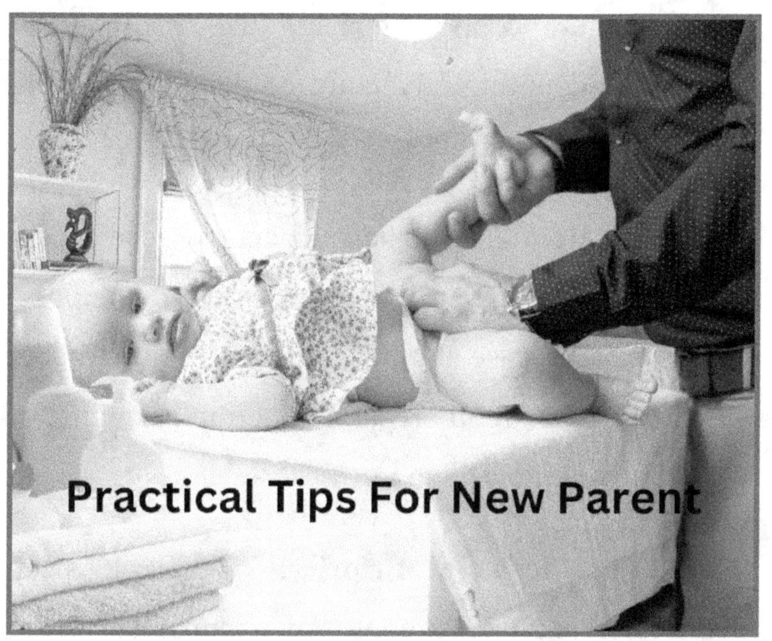

Chapter 8

Practical Tips for New Parents

To help new couples manage the thrilling but sometimes daunting adventure of parenthood, here are a variety of helpful pointers.

1. Accept Help: Never be reluctant to accept help from friends and relatives. Having a support network helps ease the adjustment to motherhood, whether it is via food preparation, errand running, or providing emotional support.

2. Make Sleep a Priority: Although sleep deprivation is typical among new parents, it's crucial for your health. When your baby sleeps during the day, take turns taking naps and feeding at night with your spouse.

3. Create Routines: Since babies do best with structure, create regular eating, sleeping, and playing schedules. Regular schedules will make your infant feel safe and encourage greater sleep.

4. Talk to Your spouse: Having a child may put stress on even the most solid relationships, so make it a priority to have direct and honest conversations with your spouse. To keep your relationship solid and encouraging, talk about your emotions, worries, and duties.

5. Exercise Self-Care: Never forget to look for yourself when looking after your child. Make time for things that help you refuel and feel refreshed, including working out, reading, or hanging out with friends.

6. Trust Your Instincts: Being a parent is a high learning curve, but you should have faith in your gut feelings. When it comes to your baby's care and welfare, trust your instincts as you are the one who knows them the best.

7. Maintain Organization: To lessen stress and anxiety, maintain organization. Parenthood may be chaotic. To keep track of appointments, deadlines, and projects, use calendars, to-do lists, and apps.

8. Get Ready for Outings: Taking a baby out involves planning and preparation. Stow away necessities like extra clothes, wipes, diapers, and feeding materials in a diaper bag. When organizing excursions, take the weather and your baby's routine into account.

9. Spend Time Rubbing: Rubbing, petting, and making eye contact with your infant to strengthen your relationship. Strong attachments and the promotion of emotional growth depend on these times of connection.

10. Develop Your Patience: Being a parent calls for patience, particularly when you're angry or tired. If you need to gather yourself, take a few deep breaths, count to 10, or take a step back.

11. Acknowledge Imperfections: Acknowledging imperfections and letting go of perfectionism are common aspects of parenthood. Recognize that mistakes will happen sometimes and that's acceptable. Just concentrate on giving it your all. Accept the flaws and uncertainty that come with being a parent, and always keep in mind that you're doing the best you can for your child.

12. Remain Informed: Remain up to date on safety regulations, child development theories, and parenting techniques. Keep abreast of healthcare guidelines, and when in doubt, seek counsel from trustworthy sources.

13. Celebrate Your Baby's Milestones: Honor every baby's accomplishment, no matter how little. Every developmental milestone—from their first grin to their first steps—is an occasion to celebrate and take stock of your baby's progress.

14. Take Care of Your Connection: Despite the responsibilities of children, schedule time for your connection with your spouse. Plan dates, be honest with each other, and express gratitude for each other's parenting efforts.

15. Make Memories: Treasure the time you spend with your child and make enduring memories. Make mementos, journal, and take pictures to remember your baby's early years.

16. Develop Gratitude: Express your thankfulness for the blessing of motherhood and the happiness your child brings into your life. Consider the good things about being a parent and give thanks for the love and bond you have with your child.

17. Seek Professional Assistance if Needed: Don't be afraid to get professional assistance if you're having problems with your mental or emotional health. Speak with a therapist, counselor, or medical professional for assistance in overcoming the obstacles of motherhood.

They may provide resources, support, and direction. Remind yourself that seeking support when needed is a show of strength rather than weakness and that you are deserving of aid and support in taking care of your well-being as a parent.

Essential Baby Equipment and Supplies

Important infant supplies and equipment are necessary to assist parents care for their babies and ease the adjustment to becoming parents. Having the appropriate equipment and supplies on hand may significantly improve the comfort, safety, and well-being of both parents and newborns in everything from feeding and diapering to sleep and safety.

Here's a thorough look at the infant supplies and equipment that every parent has to think about:

Essentials of Feeding

Breast Pump: In situations when breastfeeding is not feasible, a breast pump enables nursing moms to express milk for their infants.

Bottles and Nipples: To give their infant formula or expressed breast milk, even nursing moms may need bottles and nipples.

Formula: Having formula on hand is vital for parents who decide to use it as a feeding option or who need to supplement breast milk.

Burp cloths: During feedings, these absorbent towels assist shield clothes from spit-up.

Bottle Sterilizer: Aids in ensuring that feeding utensils and bottles are completely sterilized to stop the spread of dangerous germs.

Bottle warmer: Easy to use, safe, and fast way to warm bottles to the perfect temperature for feeding.

Breastfeeding Cover: Gives nursing moms discretion and privacy while they're out in public.

Support and comfort are provided by a nursing pillow during breastfeeding or bottle-feeding sessions.

Essentials of Diapering

Diapers: Having a large assortment of diapers in different sizes, whether they are cloth or disposable, is crucial.

Wipes: For general hygiene and cleansing during diaper changes, baby wipes come in helpful.

Cream for Diaper Rash: Assists in relieving and shielding baby's skin from irritation.

Diaper Bag Organizer: Ensures that necessities like baby wipes and diapers are conveniently arranged and accessible when traveling.

Diaper Pail: Reduces smells in the nursery by offering a quick and sanitary method to get rid of used diapers.

When traveling, this small and convenient changing kit allows for easy diaper changes.

Essentials for Sleep

A baby can sleep safely and comfortably in a crib or bassinet.

Fitted Crib Sheets: To avoid dangerously loose bedding, make sure they fit snugly.

Swaddle Blankets: By simulating the tight sensation of the womb, they aid in calming and comforting babies.

Sleep Sacks: Lower the possibility of loose bedding while offering warmth and security.

A White Noise Machine: May help block out background noise and provide a relaxing atmosphere for sleeping.

A Sound Machine: May be used to play lullabies or other calming sounds to soothe and calm newborns while they sleep.

Night Light: Softly illuminates the area so that a baby may be fed or changed in the middle of the night without interrupting their sleep schedule.

Co-Sleeper Bassinet: This bassinet firmly fastens to the parent's bedside, facilitating secure and comfortable nursing and bonding throughout the night.

Essential Clothes:

Onesies and Bodysuits: Cozy and useful for daily use.

Sleepers/Pajamas: Cozy, soft clothing for night wear. Baby's feet should be kept warm and safe with socks and booties.

Hats and Mittens: These items shield and warm a newborn's delicate hands and head.

Baby Hangers: Keep baby's clothes in the nursery closet wrinkle-free and arranged.

Baby Laundry Detergent: It's a fragrance-free, hypoallergenic detergent designed especially for cleaning baby clothes and linens.

Essentials of Safety

Car seats are necessary for neonates to be transported in cars safely.

Baby Monitor: Enables parents to keep an eye on their infant's security and health, particularly while they're asleep.

Childproofing Supplies: To baby-proof the house as it grows more mobile, get outlet covers, cabinet locks, and safety gates.

Covered Outlet Plugs: Keep little hands from reaching electrical outlets and possible dangers.

Cordless Window Blinds: Provide a secure sleeping environment for infants by removing the possibility of strangling from hanging cables.

Install safety gates with locks at the top and bottom of stairs or entrances to prevent your infant from entering dangerous locations.

Essentials for Health and Hygiene

Infant Bathtub: Offers a cozy and secure space for infant bathing.

Baby Wash and Shampoo: Gentle products designed especially for a baby's delicate skin and scalp.

Gentle Towels & Washcloths: Ideal for a baby's sensitive skin.

An Electronic Thermometer: It is necessary for tracking a baby's temperature and identifying fever.

Baby Nail File: Provides a soft substitute for nail clippers when it comes to shaping and smoothing a baby's nails. To stop a baby from scratching, use nail clippers or scissors.

Nasal Aspirator: Especially during colds or congestion, this device helps remove mucus from a baby's nasal passages to facilitate breathing.

Gentle Laundry Stain Remover: Effectively removes stubborn stains from baby's clothes and linens; no harsh chemicals or allergens.

Essentials for Travel

A Stroller: Offers a practical means of carrying a baby whether out on walks or doing errands.

Car Window Shades: Protect your infant from the sun's glare and ultraviolet radiation while you're driving.

Travel Diaper Changing Kit: Convenient and lightweight for changing diapers when driving, using a stroller, or flying.

Car Seat Travel Bag: Prevents scuffs and stains on automobile seats while stored or transported by air.

Essentials of Play and Development

A Play Mat: Gives a baby a cozy, secure area to explore and play.

Teethers and Rattles: Assist in invigorating a baby's senses and relieving teething pain.

Books: For early reading experiences, board books with straightforward drawings and vibrant colors work well.

Activity Gym: Offers engaging games and stimulation to enhance a baby's growing motor abilities and senses.

Essentials of Nursing and Feeding

Introducing solid meals to a baby requires the use of a high chair or booster seat.

Baby Bowls and Spoons: These are sized and designed to fit a baby's tiny lips and hands.

Bibs: Assist in shielding baby clothes from stains and food spills.

A Breastfeeding Pillow: Offers comfort and support during nursing sessions.

Nursing pads: These are absorbent pads that are placed inside bras to stop leaks and keep clothes dry in between feedings.

Essentials for Comfort

Pacifiers: They soothe and calm a baby in between meals.

Stylish and Cozy Nursing Chair: Offers a pleasant and supportive setting choice for nursing or bottle-feeding sessions.

Postpartum Support Belt: Promotes comfort and aids in postpartum recovery by providing mild compression and support to the lower back and abdomen.

The Wellness Tracker App: Allows parents to easily monitor their baby's growth milestones, eating, sleeping patterns, and diaper changes from the comfort of their smartphone.

Establishing a Daily Schedule with Your Infant

Establishing structure, predictability, and consistency in your everyday life as a couple requires that you and your infant have a routine. A well-thought-out routine fosters good sleep patterns and development lessens stress and anxiety, and increases security for both you and your child. Here's a detailed look at how to set up a daily schedule that works for you and your infant:

Recognize Your Baby's Developmental Stage: Knowing your baby's developmental stage and specific demands is the first step in establishing a daily routine. When compared to older babies and toddlers, newborns have altered sleep, eating, and play routines. When organizing your daily routine, take into account things like your baby's age, feeding schedule, sleep habits, and developmental milestones.

Establish Feeding Times: Considering your baby's age and nutritional requirements, schedule regular feeding times throughout the day. Although older babies may eventually start to have longer stretches between feedings, newborns often eat every two to three hours. You may include breastfeeding or bottle-feeding sessions into your baby's everyday routine to provide them with nutrients as well as chances to interact and bond.

Include Play and Interactive Time: Give your infant time to engage in play and interactive activities that will help them grow physically, mentally, and emotionally. Play games, sensory play, tummy time, music and movement, and other age-appropriate activities that promote exploration and discovery. Provide your baby with plenty of chances for hugging, chatting, singing, and making eye contact to enhance the parent-child link and awaken their senses.

Include Outdoor Time: To expose your infant to natural light, fresh air, and the sights and sounds of the outdoors, try to include some outdoor time into your daily schedule. Enjoy long strolls with the stroller, hang out in the backyard or neighborhood park, or just cuddle up on a blanket in the sun.

Spending time outside gives your infant important sensory experiences, encourages physical exercise, and stimulates their senses.

Schedule Meals and Snacks: Once your baby starts eating solid meals, be sure to include regular meals and snack times in your daily schedule. Provide a range of wholesome meals, promote self-feeding, and let them experiment with tastes and textures. During mealtimes, gather as a family to foster social contact and bonding while modeling good eating habits. To best suit your baby's requirements, adjust your schedule based on signs such as changes in behavior, mood, food, or sleep habits.

Chapter *9*

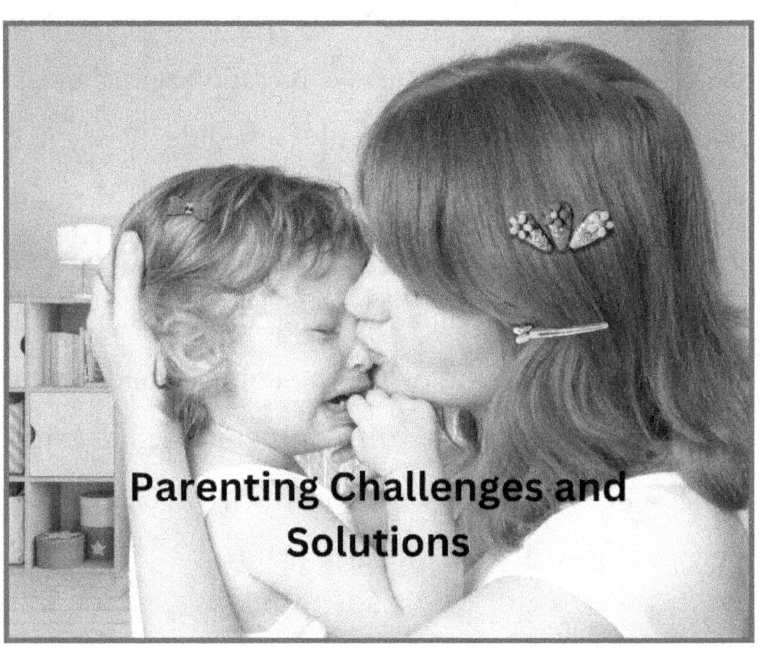

Chapter 9

Parenting Challenges and Solutions

Every parent has challenges along the road, from handling behavioral problems to negotiating developmental milestones. However, these difficulties may be solved with perseverance, understanding, and practical methods. This is a thorough overview of typical parenting problems and possible fixes:

1. Conduct Control

Challenge: Parents may find it difficult and unpleasant to handle their children's tantrums, disobedience, or other difficult behaviors.

Solution: Use positive disciplinary strategies including redirection, positive reinforcement, and rational consequences. Also, create appropriate limits and communicate expectations for conduct. To assist your kid in navigating their emotions, provide an example of polite communication and problem-solving techniques and show empathy and compassion.

2. Interaction and Formation

Challenge: When your kid gets older and starts to express their independence, it may be difficult to establish open and effective communication with them.

Solution: Provide chances for deep dialogue and quality time spent with one another. Encourage your kid to express themselves in a safe, accepting setting by actively listening to their ideas and emotions and validating their experiences. Establish a good example for polite communication and dispute resolution, and place a high value on strengthening the link between parents and children via shared interests and experiences.

3. Establishing Limits and Boundaries

Challenge: It may be difficult for parents to strike a balance between their children's demand for independence and autonomy and their need to establish rules and boundaries.

Solution: Set consistent, enforceable, age-appropriate, and unambiguous limits. When it's feasible, include your youngster in the decision-making process by explaining the rationale behind the rules and penalties. When your kid is learning to negotiate boundaries and make responsible decisions, be fair but firm in your approach and provide direction and support.

4. Controlling Technology Use and Screen Time

Challenge: In the current digital era, when screens are becoming more and more common in children's lives, setting limits on screen time and controlling technology usage may be difficult.

Solution: Clearly define expectations and guidelines for screen time, including use restrictions, acceptable material guidelines, and times or zones that are off-limits to screens. Set a good example for others by avoiding unhealthy screen use and supporting more creative or outdoor-oriented hobbies or play. Manage and monitor your child's online behavior using parental controls and monitoring tools. Have regular, honest discussions with them on responsible digital citizenship and online safety.

5. Conflict and Rivalry Among Siblings

Challenge: Families with many children often experience sibling rivalry and conflict, which causes friction and strife between siblings.

Solution: Encourage collaboration, empathy, and conflict resolution techniques to build healthy sibling relationships. Siblings should be encouraged to share their thoughts and emotions, and their experiences should be validated without taking sides. Instruct siblings in problem-solving techniques including compromise, bargaining, and sharing responsibilities. Additionally, provides them with chances to interact and cooperate via common interests and experiences.

6. Balance and Time Management

Challenge: Parents may feel overburdened and overextended while juggling the demands of employment, domestic duties, and family life.

Solution: Make self-care a priority and create a positive work-life balance by defining boundaries, assigning responsibilities, and using time management techniques. Establish plans and habits that emphasize spending quality time with your family and arrange time for self-relaxing and rejuvenating activities. Know when to say no to unimportant commitments and duties, and when you need help, reach out to friends, family, or experts.

7. Handling Burnout and Stress

Challenge: Being a parent can be emotionally and physically taxing, which may result in stress, burnout, and feelings of being inadequate or worn out.

Solution: Engage in activities that encourage relaxation, stress alleviation, and emotional resilience as a kind of self-care and prioritize your well-being. When you need it, take pauses and ask your friends, partner, or support groups for help. To handle stress, engage in mindfulness, meditation, or relaxation exercises. Recognizing when seeking professional assistance for mental health issues may be helpful.

8. Adaptability and Flexibility

Challenge: Managing unforeseen obstacles and situational changes as a parent calls for flexibility and adaptation.

Solution: Adopt a growth attitude, be creative, and address problems with resourcefulness and ingenuity. Embrace flexibility and adaptation as fundamental parenting abilities. Be flexible in your thinking, adapt your tactics as necessary, and exercise resilience when faced with challenges or disappointments. Maintain perspective and a sense of humor, and concentrate on solving issues rather than obsessing over them.

9. Looking for Resources and Assistance

Challenge: It might be challenging to ask for assistance or find resources when one feels alone or overburdened by parenting difficulties.

Solution: Seek out assistance from family members, friends, or parenting organizations that may provide understanding, motivation, and useful guidance. Use internet forums, helplines, community resources, and support services when you need further advice and support. Never be afraid to seek the advice of physicians, therapists, or other experts when you need specific help or action.

Parenting is tough, and you need to be resilient, patient, and open to learning and developing with your kid. You may overcome challenges and create a strong and supportive family dynamic that promotes development, resilience, and respect for one another by taking a proactive and upbeat attitude, asking for help when you need it, and placing a high value on connection and communication. Keep in mind that every parent has difficulties along the way, you are not experiencing it alone.

Managing Nighttime Wakings and Sleep Regression

Parents may find it difficult to deal with their children's sleep regression and overnight awakenings, but by comprehending the reasons and putting good sleep practices into practice, they may manage these phases more skillfully. A thorough approach to managing sleep regression and nightly awakenings may be found here:

Understanding Sleep Regression

An infant or toddler's sleep habits may temporarily be disrupted by sleep regression, which is often characterized by numerous overnight awakenings, trouble settling asleep, or shorter naps. Sleep regressions usually happen around 4 months, 8–10 months, 12 months, 18 months, and 2 years of age, or at predicted developmental milestones. These times are often linked to routine changes, teething, developmental leaps, and growth spurts.

Causes of Sleep Regression

- **Growth Spurts:** As your child's body and brain adjust to new milestones, rapid physical or cognitive growth may cause sleep patterns to be disrupted.

- **Teething:** Pain during teething may make it uncomfortable at night and increase the number of times you wake up throughout the night.

- **Developmental Milestones:** Developing new abilities or accomplishing developmental milestones like walking or crawling might cause restlessness or an increase in activity at night.

- **Shifts in Routine:** Sleep habits might be disturbed by adjustments to the daily routine, travel, or life changes like beginning childcare or relocating to a new place.

Developing Healthy Sleep Routines

- **Reliable Bedtime Schedule:** Create a relaxing bedtime schedule that lets your kids know when it's time to unwind and get ready for bed. This might include doing things like taking a warm bath, reading, or softly rocking.

- **Consistent Sleep Environment:** Establish a peaceful, dark, and cozy sleeping environment. To encourage sound sleep, use white noise generators, blackout curtains, and cozy bedding.

- **Daytime Sleep Schedule:** Make sure your kids receive enough sleep throughout the day to avoid becoming overtired, which may make their overnight awakenings worse. Maintain a regular sleep pattern and give age-appropriate wake windows priority.

- **Promote Self-Soothing:** If your kid wakes up during the night, teach them self-soothing skills to help them go back to sleep on their own. This may be providing a cuddly toy or comfort item, using mild sleep training techniques, or sticking to a regular bedtime schedule.

Handling Night Wakings

- **React Consistently:** When your kid wakes up in the middle of the night, comfort and reassure them constantly. Provide comfort, but refrain from engaging in extended or stimulating activities that might exacerbate sleep disturbances.

- **Check for Discomfort:** Take quick care of your child's needs if they are in discomfort due to sickness, teething, or other physical problems. If required, provide comfort measures, painkillers, or medical treatment.

- **Steer clear of Sleep Associations:** Take care not to establish sleep associations that depend on outside assistance or parental supervision to fall asleep. To become less reliant on other sources of comfort, help your kid develop the ability to self-soothe and go to sleep on their own.

Sustaining Self-Care as a Parent

- **Put Your Sleep First:** As a parent, make sure that your sleep and well-being come first. Take turns waking up throughout the night with your spouse, or think about getting a reliable caregiver to assist so that you can get the restorative sleep you need.

- **Seek Support:** If you're feeling overburdened or worn out, don't be afraid to ask friends, family, or medical experts for assistance. A doctor or sleep expert may provide useful information and comfort, such as joining parent support groups.

- **Be Patient and Persistent:** Keep in mind that sleep regressions are transient and usually go away on their own. When your kid acclimates to new routines and developmental milestones, their sleep patterns should settle, so be patient and persistent in your approach.

- **Remain adaptive and flexible:** Adapting your tactics to suit your child's evolving sleep requirements and developmental phases.

You may assist your kid traverse these issues more easily and encourage peaceful and restorative sleep for the whole family by learning the reasons for sleep regression and nightly awakenings and have patience as your child's sleep habits will eventually get better.

Handling Picky Eating and Challenges at Meals

It may be difficult for parents to deal with fussy eating and mealtime challenges, but with perseverance, consistency, and imagination, you can help your kid develop healthy eating habits and have a good mealtime experience. The following useful advice will help you deal with fussy eaters and mealtime challenges:

1. Have Reasonable Expectations: Recognize that fussy eating is a typical stage of childhood growth and maybe something your kid outgrows in due course. Mealtime anxiety and resistance may be caused by exerting excessive pressure on your kid to clear their plate or consume certain items.

2. Offer a Variety of meals: Even if your kid first rejects them, introduce a broad range of meals early on and keep offering them regularly. As your child's taste grows, encourage experimentation and discovery with a variety of flavors, textures, and colors.

3. Serve as an Example: Kids tend to imitate their parents' eating habits, so set a good example by including a range of nutrient-dense foods in your meals. When feasible, eat meals as a family and show excitement in trying new dishes.

4. Include Your Kid: Give your kid responsibility by letting them help with grocery shopping, menu planning, and cooking. Allow children to help with basic chores like washing produce or mixing recipes, or let them choose fruits and veggies at the grocery store.

5. Establish a Positive Mealtime Environment: Reduce distractions and emphasize connection and discussion to make mealtimes fun and laid back. Refrain from using food as a reward or a weapon at mealtimes.

6. Serve Meals in a Family Style: Let your kids help themselves with meals and decide how much of each item to place on their plate. In addition to fostering self-regulation of hunger and fullness signals, this fosters autonomy.

7. Provide Regular Meal and Snack Times: To assist control your child's appetite and avoid excessive hunger or grazing throughout the day, set up a regular meal and snack plan. To fill up the gaps in your appetite and provide you energy between meals, offer wholesome snacks.

8. Make Nutritious Foods Accessible: Stock your house with easily accessible and visually appealing nutritious foods, such as lean meats, whole grains, and chopped fruits and veggies. Restrict the availability of processed meals, sugar-filled drinks, and sugary snacks.

9. Get Creative with Presentation: Present meals in entertaining and attractive ways to make them more desirable to your youngster. Utilize cookie cutters to creatively shape fruits and veggies, or arrange food in animal or facial forms on the dish.

10. Offer Options Within Limits: To help your kid feel in charge and independent, offer them options at mealtimes. At each meal, provide two or three alternatives; nevertheless, make sure that every selection is wholesome and agreeable to you as the parent.

11. Promote Exploration: Let your kids try new foods at their own pace, free from force or pressure. Present modest samples of new dishes alongside well-known classics and acknowledge little accomplishments and advancements.

12. Keep at It: Handling fussy eating is a gradual process that calls for perseverance and patience. Even if things go slowly, stick to your plan and fight the temptation to give in to power battles over food.

13. Don't Force or Bribe: Refrain from employing coercive methods or incentives to get your kid to eat, since this may cause them to associate food negatively and develop resistance. Give them encouragement, compliments, and positive reinforcement instead, if they try new foods or eat healthily.

14. Seek Professional Assistance if Needed: You should think about seeing a physician, registered dietitian, or feeding therapist if your child's fussy eating habits have a negative influence on their development, nutritional intake, or general well-being. They may provide tailored suggestions and methods to meet the unique requirements of your kid.

You may assist manage fussy eating and mealtime conflicts while encouraging your kid to have a happy and healthy connection with food by putting these helpful recommendations into practice. You can help your kid develop lifetime habits of eating healthily and appreciating a broad range of foods if you put in the necessary time and effort.

Chapter 10

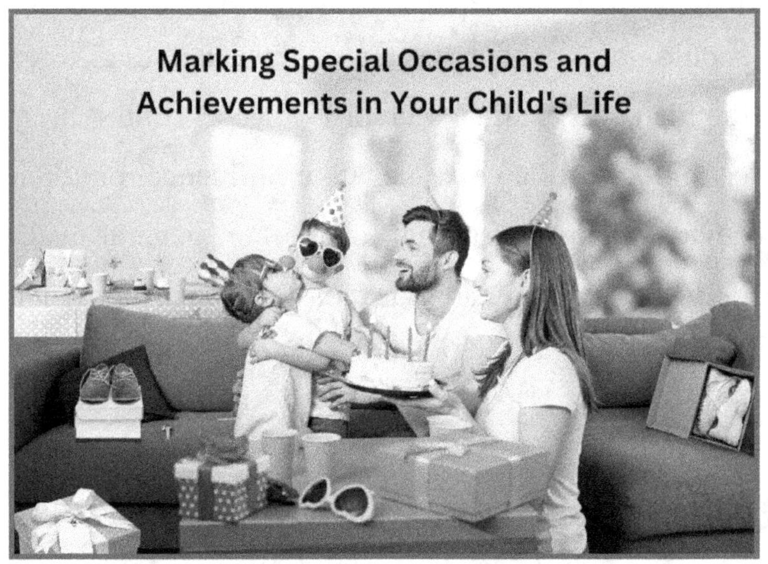

Chapter 10

Marking Special Occasions and Achievements in Your Child's Life

A vital aspect of parenting is commemorating milestones and holidays in your kid's life. These activities provide you the chance to make priceless memories and help your child feel proud, self-assured, and like they belong. Here are some ideas for making your child's milestones, birthdays, graduations, and personal achievements special and unforgettable:

1. Birthdays: A child's birthday commemorates another year of life and memories, and it's an opportunity to honor your child's development and accomplishments. Organize unique events or excursions that suit your child's interests and preferences. Some ideas include a family adventure, a day trip to their favorite place, or a themed party. Let your kids help organize the party by letting them choose the birthday celebration's theme, events, and invite list. Establish customs and routines that add a particular touch to birthday celebrations.

Some ideas include having breakfast in bed on important occasions, taking family photos, or penning sincere notes to your kid.

2. Stages and Achievements: Congratulate your kid on all of his or her accomplishments, like learning to ride a bike, picking up a new talent, or hitting a sporting or scholastic benchmark. Congratulate your youngster on their efforts and advancements, highlighting their tenacity, willpower, and fortitude. Arrange unique events or trips to honor noteworthy accomplishments. Some ideas include a modest celebration with friends and family, a day trip to a particular location, or a family meal at their favorite restaurant.

To preserve your child's milestones and accomplishments, assemble a scrapbook or memory box with pictures, keepsakes, and encouraging words.

3. Graduations and Promotions: The fruits of hard effort and devotion, graduations, and promotions are important turning points in your child's academic or personal path. Whether it's a graduation ceremony, a promotion ceremony, or a special family supper, plan events or ceremonies to celebrate your child's achievements. Include loved ones in the festivities by extending an invitation to them to partake in the happiness and excitement around your child's accomplishment.

To mark the event, think about giving your kid a sentimental present or symbol of gratitude, such as a customized memento, a unique experience, or a piece of jewelry.

4. Personal Achievements: Congratulate your kid on all of their achievements, whether it's playing in a school play, winning a sporting event, or taking part in a community service initiative. Show your support and encouragement by being there at your child's activities and performances. Cheer them on from the sidelines and take joy in their accomplishments. Acknowledge and commend your kid for his or her efforts and accomplishments, stressing the need for tenacity, fortitude, and cooperation.

Showcase your child's abilities and accomplishments by placing their artwork, diplomas, or trophies in a visible area of your house. This will inspire pride and success in them.

5. Gratitude and Reflection: Spend some time thinking back on your child's successes and turning points, and give thanks for all of their hard work, devotion, and tenacity. Show your appreciation for your child's existence and the happiness and contentment they provide to your family. Encourage your kid to think back on their successes and turning points to help them feel proud of and confident in their talents.

Utilize milestones and special events to show your kid how much you care and how much you appreciate them. This will help them understand how important it is to celebrate accomplishments and acknowledge hard work.

6. Making Lasting Memories: Document the happiness and excitement of these times by capturing and preserving memories of noteworthy events and accomplishments via pictures, films, or writing. Make a scrapbook or memory book with pictures, keepsakes, and personal remarks to honor your child's accomplishments and milestones. Take some time to go over these memories with your family, remembering former events and anniversaries and thinking back on your child's development.

To give your kid a feeling of agency and control over their life experiences, encourage them to create their traditions and memories.

By commemorating milestones and important events in your child's life, you provide chances for development, happiness, and connection that they will remember for years to come. These occasions mark significant turning points in their life and provide chances to build enduring memories and reinforce family relationships.

Chapter *11*

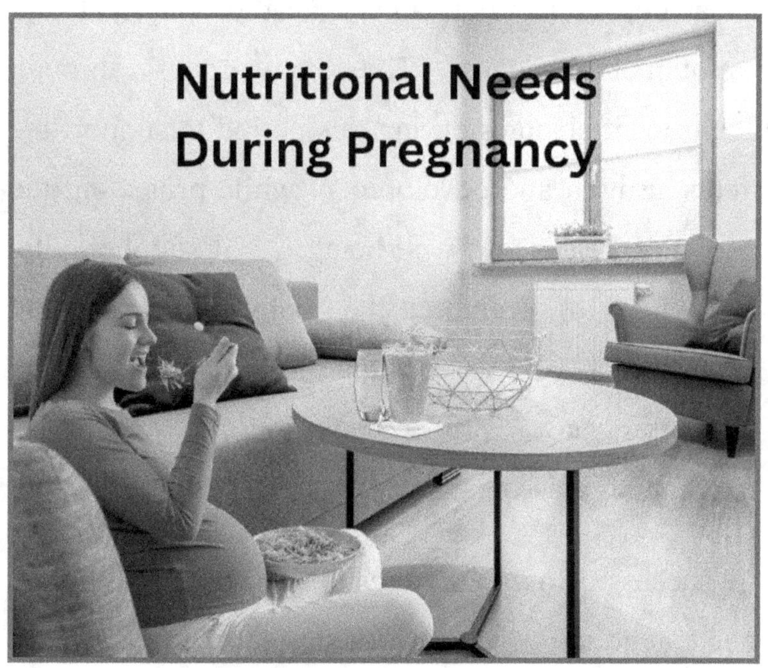

Chapter 11

Nutritional Needs During Pregnancy

Pregnancy is a voyage of transformation full of pleasure, excitement, and a host of physical and emotional changes. The body goes through significant changes during this period to support the fetus' growth and development while protecting the mother's health and well-being. As it supplies vital nutrients to promote the baby's growth and development and to keep the mother healthy during the pregnancy, proper nutrition is critical in facilitating these changes.

A successful pregnancy result depends on knowing the unique dietary requirements throughout pregnancy. Let's examine the essential nutrients needed in each trimester in-depth, along with dietary suggestions and helpful hints for achieving these requirements.

First Trimester

The baby develops quickly during the first trimester as its main organs and systems start to take shape. The mother's dietary requirements are increased at this stage to support the development surge. During the first trimester, some important nutrients to pay attention to are:

Folic Acid: Due to its critical function in preventing neural tube disorders like spina bifida, folic acid is perhaps the most important vitamin during the first trimester. Pregnant women should take 600–800 mcg of folic acid per day. Citrus fruits, legumes, leafy greens, and fortified cereals are good dietary sources.

Iron: During pregnancy, iron is necessary for the creation of red blood cells and the transportation of oxygen. About 27 milligrams of iron are required daily by pregnant women to sustain the growing fetus and increase blood volume. Lean meats, chicken, fish, beans, lentils, tofu, and fortified cereals are all excellent dietary sources of iron.

Calcium: Both the mother's bone health and the development of the baby's bones and teeth depend on calcium. Aim for 1,000 mg of calcium every day if you're pregnant. Fortified plant-based substitutes and leafy greens are good sources of calcium, as are dairy products like milk, yogurt, and cheese.

Vitamin D: Vitamin D supports the immune system and bone health by collaborating with calcium. Aim for 600–800 IU (International Units) of vitamin D daily for expectant mothers. Sunlight exposure, fortified dairy products, and fatty fish (like salmon and mackerel) are good dietary sources.

Omega-3 Fatty Acids: The development of the baby's brain and vision depends on omega-3 fatty acids, especially DHA (docosahexaenoic acid). Aim for a daily intake of DHA of at least 200–300 mg for expectant mothers. Walnuts, flaxseeds, chia seeds, fatty fish (salmon, mackerel, and sardines), and supplements made of algae are good dietary sources.

Pregnant women should prioritize eating a well-balanced diet that contains a range of fruits, vegetables, whole grains, lean meats, and healthy fats in addition to these essential nutrients. During the first trimester, it's also critical to stay hydrated by drinking plenty of water, particularly if morning sickness is evident.

Second Trimester

Pregnancy's "honeymoon phase" is typically referred to as the second trimester as many women report feeling less fatigued and sick than they usually do in the first trimester. The baby is still developing quickly at this period, and its dietary demands are still high. The following are important nutrients to pay attention to in the second trimester:

Protein: To support the baby's growth and development as well as the mother's own tissue repair and immune system, a higher amount of protein is needed during pregnancy. Aim for around 71 grams of protein each day when pregnant. Lean meats, poultry, fish, eggs, dairy products, legumes, nuts, and seeds are all excellent dietary sources.

Fiber: During pregnancy, constipation is a typical problem that may be avoided with the use of fiber. Aim for at least 25–30 grams of fiber per day for pregnant women, coming from whole grains, fruits, vegetables, legumes, nuts, and seeds.

Vitamin C: Iron absorption, collagen formation, and immunological function all depend on vitamin C. Aim for 85 milligrams of vitamin C every day when pregnant. Citrus fruits, strawberries, kiwis, bell peppers, broccoli, and tomatoes are good dietary sources.

B vitamins: During pregnancy, B vitamins have several functions in energy metabolism, DNA synthesis, and nervous system function. These include vitamin B1 (thiamine), vitamin B2 (riboflavin), vitamin B3 (niacin), vitamin B5 (pantothenic acid), vitamin B6 (pyridoxine), vitamin B7 (biotin), vitamin B9 (folate), and vitamin B12 (cobalamin). The goal for pregnant women should be to get enough of these vitamins via a diversified diet that includes dairy products, whole grains, lean meats, leafy greens, and fortified foods.

Magnesium: Magnesium is necessary for healthy bones, muscles, and nerves. The daily goal for pregnant women should be between 350 and 360 mg of magnesium. Whole grains, legumes, nuts, seeds, leafy greens, and dairy products are examples of good dietary sources.

Pregnant women should concentrate on healthily gaining weight and continuing to exercise throughout the second trimester since these variables might affect the health of the mother and the result of the pregnancy.

Third Trimester

The baby grows and develops quickly throughout the third trimester, and the mother has growing physical pain during this time as well. During this period, the mother's health and well-being, the baby's development, and the preparation for labor and delivery are all dependent on proper nutrition. The following are important nutrients to pay attention to in the third trimester:

Omega-3 Fatty Acids: Throughout the third trimester, the development of the baby's brain and eyes is supported by the consumption of omega-3 fatty acids. Aim for a daily intake of DHA of 200–

300 mg for expectant mothers, consuming it from foods including walnuts, flaxseeds, chia seeds, fatty fish, and algae-based supplements.

Calcium and vitamin D: These two nutrients are still crucial for the mother's bone health and the development of the baby's bones throughout the third trimester. The daily goals for pregnant women should remain to get 600–800 IU of vitamin D and 1,000 mg of calcium from diets that include dairy products, fortified plant-based foods, lipid-laden seafood, and exposure to sunshine.

Iron: To sustain the baby's growing blood volume and shield the mother against iron-deficiency anemia, iron requirements remain high throughout the third trimester. The daily target for iron intake for expectant mothers is about 27 milligrams, which may be obtained from foods including lean meats, chicken, fish, beans, lentils, tofu, and fortified cereals.

Protein: The mother's immune system and tissue healing, as well as the baby's growth and development, depend on her body obtaining enough protein throughout the third trimester. The recommended daily intake of protein for expectant mothers is 71 grams, which may be obtained from foods including lean meats, chicken, fish, eggs, dairy products, legumes, nuts, and seeds.

Fiber: To avoid constipation and foster digestive health, fiber is still crucial throughout the third trimester. Aiming for at least 25–30 grams of fiber per day from whole grains, fruits, vegetables, legumes, nuts, and seeds is still a good goal for pregnant women.

Pregnant women should prioritize getting enough water throughout the day to be hydrated in addition to these essential nutrients. Maintaining amniotic fluid levels, promoting the baby's growth and development, and avoiding issues from dehydration all depend on getting enough water.

Understanding Foodborne Illness

Pregnant women should be aware of the following specific dietary recommendations and concerns in addition to making sure their basic nutritional requirements are met.

During pregnancy, when the health and well-being of the mother and the unborn child are at risk, food safety is very important. We will cover all the bases in this extensive talk on food safety, including possible hazards, proper food handling and preparation practices, and methods to reduce the chance of contracting a foodborne disease while pregnant.

When hazardous bacteria, viruses, parasites, or toxins are present in food, it may lead to foodborne sickness, often known as food poisoning. Foodborne illnesses may cause anything from minor gastrointestinal distress to severe dehydration, organ failure, and perhaps fatality. Foodborne illnesses are more common in pregnant women because of immune system alterations, hormonal changes, and possible effects on the growing fetus.

Common Sources of Foodborne Illness

Foodborne illness may be caused by several things, such as handling food incorrectly, not cooking or storing it properly, cross-contamination, and eating raw or undercooked food. Typical origins of foodborne disease consist of:

Raw or Undercooked Meats and Seafood: Bacteria that may cause illness, such as salmonella and E. coli, can be found in raw or undercooked meats, poultry, seafood, and eggs. Listeria, toxoplasma, and coli. Pregnant women and their unborn children are in danger from these germs, which may cause severe sickness.

Unpasteurized Dairy Goods: Dairy goods that have not been pasteurized, such as milk, cheese, and yogurt, may contain dangerous germs like listeria that may lead to foodborne illnesses. Pasteurized dairy products are the better choice for expectant mothers to lower the danger of infection.

Raw Fruits and Vegetables: During cultivation, harvesting, processing, or handling, raw fruits and vegetables may get infected with bacteria or parasites. Before eating, all fruits and vegetables must be well-cleaned under running water to get rid of germs, dirt, and pesticide residues.

Cross-Contamination: When dangerous germs from raw foods come into touch with prepared foods or surfaces used in food preparation, cross-contamination takes place. Using distinct cutting boards, cutlery, and food storage containers for raw and cooked meals is crucial to preventing cross-contamination. You should also properly wash your hands after handling raw food.

Improper Food Storage: Storing perishable foods improperly may encourage the development of germs and raise the risk of contracting a foodborne disease. Perishable goods should be stored at the proper temperature and quickly refrigerated to preserve freshness and safety.

Safe Food Handling and Preparation Guidelines

It's important to use proper food handling and preparation techniques to reduce the chance of foodborne disease during pregnancy. Here are some pointers to remember:

Wash Your Hands Thoroughly: Before and after handling food, using the toilet, changing diapers, or contacting animals, wash your hands thoroughly for at least 20 seconds with soap and water.

Clean Surfaces and Utensils: To avoid cross-contamination, wash cutting boards, counters, utensils, and surfaces used for food preparation with hot, soapy water after each use.

Keep Raw and Cooked Foods Separate: To avoid cross-contamination, keep raw and cooked foods in different cutting boards, utensils, and food storage containers.

Cook Foods to Safe Temperatures: To destroy dangerous germs, cook foods, particularly meats, poultry, shellfish, and eggs, to safe internal temperatures. To make sure food is cooked to the right temperature, use a food thermometer.

Store Perishable Goods in the Refrigerator: To prevent bacterial development and preserve freshness, store perishable goods including meat, poultry, fish, eggs, dairy products, and leftovers in the refrigerator as soon as possible.

Safely Thaw Meals: To stop dangerous germs from growing, thaw frozen meals in the refrigerator, microwave, or cold water bath rather than at room temperature.

Foods High in Risk: Steer clear of foods high in risk, including raw or undercooked meats, poultry, shellfish, eggs, dairy products that haven't been pasteurized, raw sprouts, and prepared meals that have been left out at room temperature for a long time.

Reducing the Risks of Pregnancy

To reduce the chance of contracting a foodborne disease and safeguard your health and the unborn child's, pregnant women should take extra measures. Pregnant women should consider the following particular recommendations:

Pregnant women should abstain from several high-risk items, including raw or undercooked meats, poultry, shellfish, eggs, unpasteurized dairy products, raw sprouts, and potentially contaminated ready-to-eat meals.

Be Aware of Food Safety When Eating Out: Pregnant women should steer clear of high-risk meals that might increase their chance of contracting a foodborne disease and instead pick reliable eateries that adhere to stringent food safety regulations.

Limiting Specific Foods and Substances: The mother's and the unborn child's health and well-being need to limit specific foods and substances throughout pregnancy. Because pregnant women are more sensitive to possible dangers than other people, it is important to minimize the chance of difficulties and encourage a positive pregnancy result by abstaining from dangerous drugs. Let's discuss what foods and drugs should be restricted or avoided during pregnancy, the rationale behind these suggestions, and how to make healthful decisions.

Alcohol: The most well-recognized advice for expectant mothers is to abstain from alcohol completely. Fetal alcohol spectrum disorders (FASDs) are a group of birth abnormalities and developmental problems that may result from alcohol use during pregnancy. Alcohol can pass the placenta and affect the developing infant.

Physical anomalies, intellectual impairments, behavioral and learning issues, and development limitations are a few examples of these. It is advised that pregnant women refrain from consuming alcohol entirely to safeguard the health of their unborn child since there is currently no established safe amount of alcohol intake during pregnancy.

Coffee: Although it is generally thought that moderate caffeine intake is safe during pregnancy, excessive caffeine consumption has been linked to higher risks of miscarriage, preterm delivery, low birth weight, and other problems. Consequently, it is advised that expectant mothers limit their daily caffeine consumption to a maximum of 200–300 mg, or around one to two cups of coffee.

It is crucial to remember that caffeine may also be present in tea, soda, energy drinks, chocolate, and certain pharmaceuticals. As such, it is necessary to monitor your total intake of caffeine from all sources.

Fish with a High Mercury: Some fish species have high levels of mercury, a hazardous element that may damage an unborn child's developing brain system. Sharks, swordfish, king mackerel, and tilefish are among the high-mercury fish that expectant mothers should stay away from or consume in moderation. Rather, they need to choose less mercury-containing options including salmon, shrimp, pollock, catfish, and canned light tuna. It is important to remember that canned albacore tuna and tuna steak have greater mercury content and should only be eaten in moderation.

Seafood With Raw or Undercooked Meats: Eggs, poultry, shellfish, and raw or undercooked meats increase the risk of contracting a foodborne disease from bacteria, parasites, or viruses such as toxoplasma, salmonella, or listeria. Preterm delivery, stillbirth, miscarriage, and serious disease in the unborn child are just a few of the issues that may arise from these illnesses, which can be especially harmful during pregnancy.

Pregnant women should avoid eating raw or undercooked eggs, unpasteurized dairy products, and raw or undercooked sprouts to lower their chances of contracting a foodborne disease. They should also make sure that all meats and seafood are cooked through to the required internal temperature.

Unpasteurized dairy products and soft cheeses: Unpasteurized dairy products including soft cheeses like feta, brie, camembert, queso blanco, and queso fresco may have dangerous germs like listeria that may lead to foodborne illnesses. Pregnant women should prefer pasteurized dairy products and steer clear of soft cheeses and unpasteurized dairy completely to lower their risk of listeriosis. When eating out or buying prepared meals, it's critical to read food labels and find out if dairy products have undergone pasteurization.

Raw Sprout: Alfalfa, clover, radish, and mung bean sprouts are among the raw sprouts that have been connected to foodborne disease outbreaks brought on by bacteria like E. and salmonella. Coli. Sprouts may get contaminated by these bacteria while they are developing and may be difficult to fully eradicate. Pregnant women should choose cooked sprouts, which are safe to consume, to lower their chance of contracting a foodborne disease.

Artificial Sweeteners: It is advised to stay away from certain artificial sweeteners including saccharin, cyclamate, and acesulfame-K while pregnant since they may be harmful to the unborn child. While it's widely accepted that consuming aspartame, sucralose, and stevia in moderation is safe, it's important to speak with your healthcare professional to be sure these sweeteners are acceptable for your particular health condition before taking them during pregnancy.

Meals Plan During Pregnancy

Meals Plan During Pregnancy

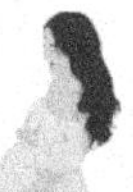

	Breakfast	Lunch	Dinner	Fruits
M	Veggie omelette with whole grain toast	Spinach and quinoa salad with grilled shrimp	Chicken and vegetable kebabs with whole wheat couscous	Sliced kiwi and strawberries
T	Whole grain toast with almond butter and sliced banana	Quinoa tabbouleh with grilled chicken	Vegetable stir-fry with tofu and brown rice	Orange segments and pineapple chunks
W	Chickpea and vegetable stir-fry with brown rice	Mediterranean chickpea salad with cucumber and tomato	Turkey burgers with sweet potato fries and mixed greens salad	Apple slices and blueberries
Th	Veggie omelette with whole grain toast	Black bean and corn salad with avocado lime dressing	Grilled salmon with sautéed spinach and quinoa	Grapes and orange segments
F	Smoothie bowl with spinach, banana, and almond milk topped with granola	Lentil and vegetable soup with a side of whole grain bread	Baked chicken thighs with roasted Brussels sprouts and sweet potatoes	Cherry tomatoes and cucumber slices
S	Breakfast burrito with scrambled eggs, black beans, and salsa	Greek salad with grilled shrimp and whole wheat pita bread	Turkey chili with cornbread muffins	Pineapple chunks and pear slices
Su	Banana walnut muffins with a side of Greek yogurt	Quinoa and black bean salad with avocado dressing	Grilled chicken breast with roasted vegetables and couscous	Mango slices and watermelon cubes

Enjoy Your Meals...

Chapter *12*

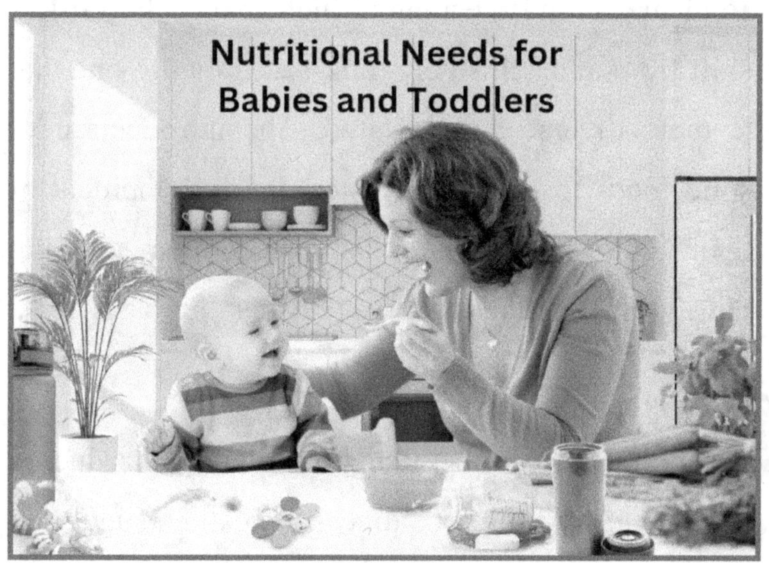

Chapter 12

Nutritional Needs for Babies and Toddlers

A baby's growth is marked by the introduction of solid meals and weaning, which marks the critical shift from an exclusively milk-based diet to one that is more diverse and textured. The introduction of solid foods to newborns fosters the development of their motor and oral skills, meets their growing nutritional demands, and establishes the basis for a lifetime of good eating habits.

We will go over the fundamentals of introducing solid meals, weaning readiness indicators, suggested feeding procedures, possible obstacles, and transitional transition tactics in this in-depth conversation.

Significance of Weaning and Solid Foods

Weaning is the process of moving from breast milk or formula to solid meals, and is a crucial developmental stage for infants. For the first six months of life, breast milk or formula supplies all the nutrients a baby needs; but, as a baby grows, solid meals must be introduced to fulfill its rising energy and nutritional needs. Additionally, important functions of solid meals include helping newborns improve their oral motor skills, encouraging self-feeding abilities, and exposing them to a wide range of flavors, textures, and tastes.

Signs of Readiness for Weaning

It's important to recognize the weaning window for your infant to facilitate a smooth transition to solid meals. Even though each kid is different, there are a few typical indicators of preparedness to watch out for:

Capacity to Sit Up: Before beginning solid meals, babies should be able to sit up with assistance and have adequate head control. This makes it easier for newborns to swallow food and reduces the risk of choking.

Loss of Tongue Thrust Reflex: Babies find it simpler to take solid meals when their tongue thrust reflex, which prompts them to push food out of their mouths with their tongues, usually goes away at six months of age.

Interest in Food: Infants who grasp food, show an interest in seeing others eat, or open their lips when given a spoon may be prepared to begin solid foods.

Enhanced Appetite: Infants may exhibit symptoms of seeking more than simply breast milk or formula and may feel hungrier in between milk feeding.

Ability to Chew or Gum-Food: Infants should be able to start chewing or gumming soft, mashed meals after being able to transfer food from the front of their mouths to the rear.

Recommended Feeding Practices

It's crucial to adhere to suggested feeding guidelines when introducing solid meals to your infant to guarantee a fun and safe experience:

Start with Single-Ingredient Meals: Start with meals that are high in iron and only include one ingredient, such as pureed fruits or vegetables or baby cereal with added iron. This enables you to recognize and keep an eye out for any possible dietary intolerances or allergies.

One New Food at a Time: When introducing new meals, do it one at a time and wait a few days before doing so again. This enables you to watch for any negative effects and spot any dietary sensitivities.

Provide a Range of Textures: As your baby's oral motor abilities advance, progressively introduce meals with thicker textures and lumpier ingredients.

Serve a range of textures, such as finely chopped meals, mashed foods, purees, and soft finger foods.

Encourage Self-Feeding: Provide finger foods and tiny, safe utensils so that your infant may explore and try self-feeding. This encourages self-control over portion sizes, independence, and fine motor abilities.

Observe Your Infant's Cues: Allow your infant to choose how much to eat by paying attention to their signs of hunger and fullness. Refrain from coercing or imposing food on your infant and have faith that they will eat enough to suit their nutritional requirements.

Keep the Feeding Environment Positive: Establish a peaceful, easygoing, and encouraging eating atmosphere that is devoid of interruptions, demands, or compulsion. Serve meals and snacks regularly and refrain from using food as a form of discipline or reward.

Possible Challenges and Solution Techniques

Parents may find it difficult to navigate the difficulties involved with weaning and introducing solid meals, but these hurdles may be successfully overcome with preparation, knowledge, and patience. Let's examine each issue in more depth and talk about potential remedies:

1. Food rejection or fussy Eating: When exposed to new foods or textures, many newborns display food rejection or fussy eating tendencies. For parents who are eager to provide their children with a healthy diet, this may be difficult.

Solution:

- Serve a range of foods. Introduce a diverse array of tastes, textures, and hues to promote experimentation and embracement of novel culinary experiences.

- **Remain patient:** It could take a few exposures for a baby to accept a new meal, so keep introducing items that the infant rejects without pressuring or forcing them.

- Serve as a role model for your child by eating meals with them and expressing your pleasure in a range of foods to inspire imitation.

- **Provide options:** Give your infant a choice between two or three nutritious foods so they can participate in mealtime decision-making.

- **Think beyond the box**: To accommodate your baby's tastes and developmental stage, provide meals in a variety of forms (such as purees, mashed potatoes, and finger foods).

2. Choking Hazard: When solid meals are introduced to newborns, there is an increased chance of choking, particularly when big, round, or hard items are served.

Solution:

- **Serve dietary-appropriate food:** Serve tiny, soft items that are easy to handle, including cooked grains, finely chopped meats, and mashed fruits and vegetables.
- **Oversee the meals:** When feeding or snacking with your baby, always keep an eye on them and stay close by in case they choke.
- Acquire knowledge about baby CPR skills to ensure you are prepared for any choking emergency.
- **Steer clear of foods high in risk:** Avoid foods that might cause choking, such as raw vegetable pieces, popcorn, hard sweets, nuts, and entire grapes.

3. Digestion Disturbance: Constipation, diarrhea, or gas are among the digestive disturbances that might sometimes result from introducing new meals.

Solution:

- **Introduce dietary items gradually:** One new meal at a time should be introduced, and you should wait a few days before introducing another to ensure there are no negative responses.
- **Present foods high in fiber:** To encourage regular bowel movements, eat a lot of foods high in fiber, such as fruits, vegetables, whole grains, and legumes.
- Drink plenty of water in between meals to keep your body hydrated and to help your digestive system.
- **Keep an eye on portion sizes:** Provide sensible serving amounts to avoid

overindulging, which may aggravate stomach issues.

4. Allergic responses: Certain foods, such as wheat, eggs, cow's milk, or peanuts, might cause allergic responses in certain newborns.

Solution:

- **Carefully introduce items that cause allergies:** One common allergenic food at a time, in modest quantities, should be introduced to ensure that no negative reactions occur.

- **Keep an eye out for allergy symptoms:** Pay close attention to any symptoms of an allergic response, such as rash, hives, swelling, vomiting, or trouble breathing. If required, get medical help.

- **Speak with a medical professional:** See a doctor or allergist for advice on introducing allergenic foods if you have a family history of food allergies or if you are concerned about your baby's potential for allergies.

Preparing Healthful Meals for Toddlers

Preparing wholesome meals for toddlers, who range in age from one to three years, is essential to promoting their general health, development, and growth. Toddlers need a balanced diet that delivers important nutrients to fuel their energy demands, boost brain development, and help them build strong bones and muscles during this time of fast growth and development.

We will cover the dietary requirements of toddlers, methods for preparing meals that are balanced, and advice for encouraging wholesome eating habits in this in-depth conversation.

Toddlers' Nutritional Needs

Toddlers' dietary requirements are different from those of older kids and babies. Toddlers need a range of nutrients to support their physical and cognitive development throughout this crucial period of growth and development. Toddlers need several essential nutrients, including:

Protein: Building and mending tissues, promoting development, and maintaining a strong immune system all depend on protein. Lean meats, poultry, fish, eggs, dairy products, legumes, tofu, and nut butter are all excellent sources of protein for toddlers.

Carbohydrates: Essential for toddlers' busy lifestyles, carbohydrates are the body's major energy source. Whole grains are great sources of complex carbohydrates that provide you with long-lasting energy. Examples of whole grains include brown rice, whole grain pasta, whole wheat bread, oats and quinoa

Healthy Fats: Hormone synthesis, nutrition absorption, and brain development all depend on healthy fats. It is recommended that toddlers be fed a diverse range of healthful fats from foods like avocados, almonds, seeds, olive oil, fatty fish (such as salmon and tuna), and nut butter.

Calcium and Vitamin D: Developing strong bones and teeth need both calcium and vitamin D. Dairy products like milk, yogurt, and cheese, as well as fortified meals like plant-based milk substitutes, are excellent sources of calcium for toddlers. In addition to fortified foods and pills, exposure to sunshine is a good source of vitamin D.

Iron: Red blood cell production and cognitive development both depend on iron. Toddlers should consume lean meats, chicken, fish, fortified cereals, beans, lentils, tofu, and dark leafy greens as well as other foods high in iron.

Fiber: Fiber helps to maintain the health of the digestive system and keeps constipation at bay. To make sure they are getting enough fiber, toddlers should eat a range of fruits, vegetables, whole grains, legumes, nuts, and seeds.

Toddlers might be reluctant to try new foods or go through stages of being picky eaters, so be patient and persistent. Even if you are first rejected while providing other dishes, have patience and keep trying. Be patient and refrain from pressing or coercing a child to eat; it may take many exposures before they are open to trying a new meal.

Meals Plan for Toddlers, (ages 1- 3 years)

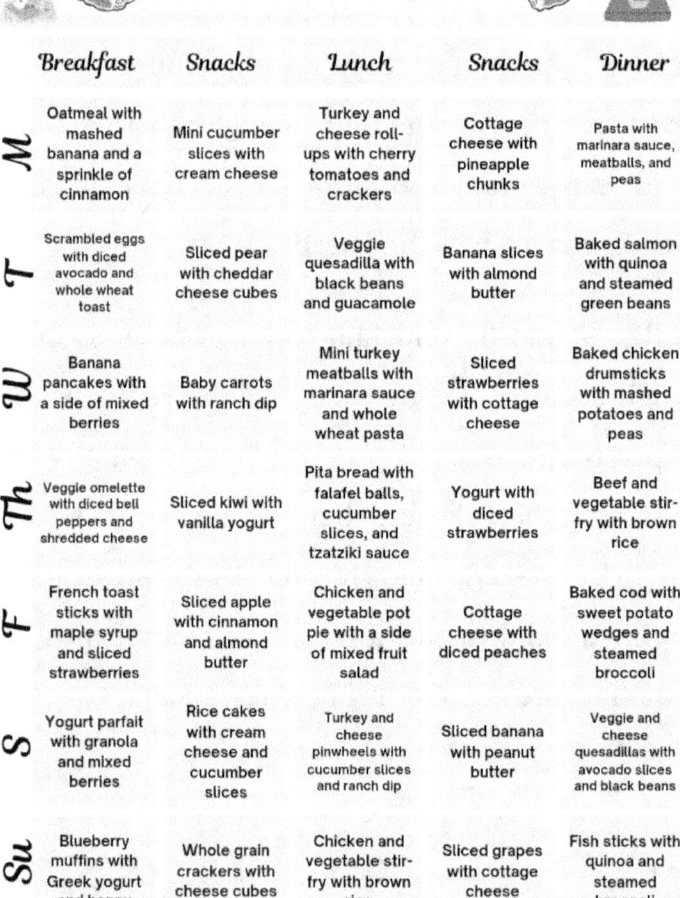

	Breakfast	Snacks	Lunch	Snacks	Dinner
M	Oatmeal with mashed banana and a sprinkle of cinnamon	Mini cucumber slices with cream cheese	Turkey and cheese roll-ups with cherry tomatoes and crackers	Cottage cheese with pineapple chunks	Pasta with marinara sauce, meatballs, and peas
T	Scrambled eggs with diced avocado and whole wheat toast	Sliced pear with cheddar cheese cubes	Veggie quesadilla with black beans and guacamole	Banana slices with almond butter	Baked salmon with quinoa and steamed green beans
W	Banana pancakes with a side of mixed berries	Baby carrots with ranch dip	Mini turkey meatballs with marinara sauce and whole wheat pasta	Sliced strawberries with cottage cheese	Baked chicken drumsticks with mashed potatoes and peas
Th	Veggie omelette with diced bell peppers and shredded cheese	Sliced kiwi with vanilla yogurt	Pita bread with falafel balls, cucumber slices, and tzatziki sauce	Yogurt with diced strawberries	Beef and vegetable stir-fry with brown rice
F	French toast sticks with maple syrup and sliced strawberries	Sliced apple with cinnamon and almond butter	Chicken and vegetable pot pie with a side of mixed fruit salad	Cottage cheese with diced peaches	Baked cod with sweet potato wedges and steamed broccoli
S	Yogurt parfait with granola and mixed berries	Rice cakes with cream cheese and cucumber slices	Turkey and cheese pinwheels with cucumber slices and ranch dip	Sliced banana with peanut butter	Veggie and cheese quesadillas with avocado slices and black beans
Su	Blueberry muffins with Greek yogurt and honey	Whole grain crackers with cheese cubes	Chicken and vegetable stir-fry with brown rice	Sliced grapes with cottage cheese	Fish sticks with quinoa and steamed broccoli

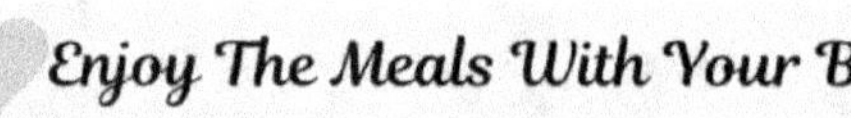

Chapter *13*

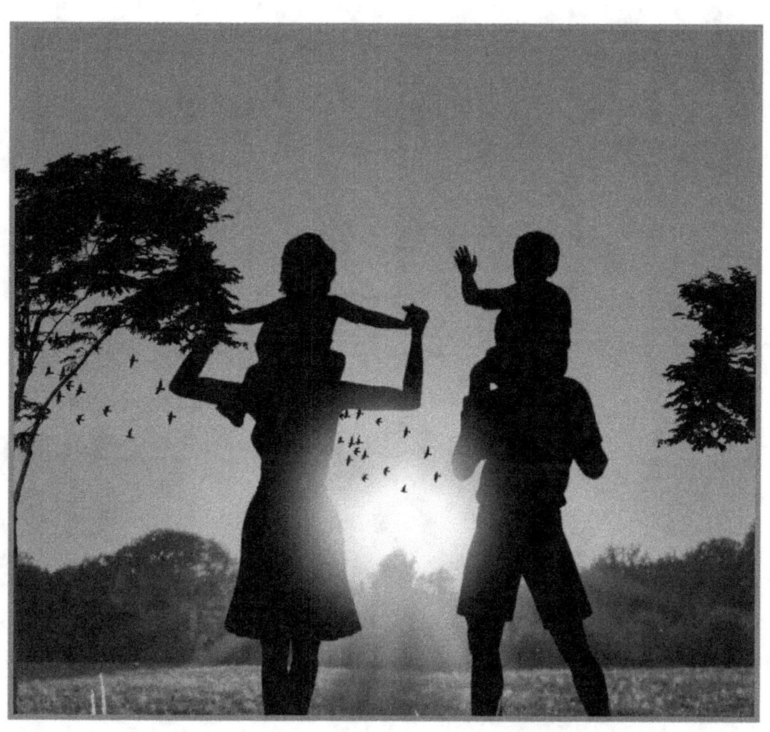

Chapter 13

Conclusion

We are excited, nervous, and maybe a little bit of both as we get ready to become parents. "Expecting Excellence in Parenting" is about enjoying the pleasures and difficulties of parenting children with optimism and confidence rather than striving for perfection. It's realizing that the mark of great parenting isn't perfection but rather a dedication to development, education, and creating deep bonds with our kids.

We've covered a lot of ground in this book on parenting, from getting ready for a baby to handling infancy to encouraging independence and creativity in early childhood. Throughout the process, we have stressed the value of flexibility, goal-setting, self-care, and fostering connections to face the unavoidable difficulties of parenting with grace and tenacity.

One of the main ideas of "Expecting Excellence in Parenting" is looking forward to the future with hope and confidence. It's about realizing that being a parent is a journey full of pleasures and pains, successes and disappointments, but one that is ultimately worthwhile to take on with bravery and optimism. Setting objectives for both ourselves and our kids and developing a flexible mentality will help us face the future with hope and confidence, knowing that we have the resources and support to overcome any obstacles that may come our way.

It's a really helpful habit to reflect on your development as a parent since it enables you to evaluate your parenting skills, pinpoint areas that need work, and acknowledge your successes along the way. Being a parent is a dynamic and constantly changing experience that is full of potential for personal development as well as pleasures and difficulties. You may improve your connection with your kid and get a deeper knowledge of yourself as a parent by pausing to think back on your experiences, choices, and interactions with them. We will go over the value of self-reflection, self-reflection techniques, and the advantages it may have on your parenting path in this in-depth conversation.

The Value of Examining Personal Development as a Parent

Self-Awareness: Taking stock of your parenting experiences and behaviors helps you become more conscious of your parenting style, values, and strengths. It enables you to recognize behavioral patterns, stressors, and responses that might affect your child-parent connection.

Personal Development: Being a parent offers a lot of chances for personal development. Thinking back on your path as a parent helps you become a more resilient, self-assured, and compassionate person by helping you learn from your experiences, difficulties, and errors.

Improved Relationship Between Parent and Child: Self-reflection helps you better understand your child's needs, temperament, and developmental stage so you can react to them patiently, empathetically, and sensitively. It creates a loving, caring connection that fortifies the link between you and your kid.

Effective Communication: You may find strategies to strengthen your communication abilities and promote polite, honest, and open discourse by thinking back on your interactions with your kid and your communication style. Building trust, settling disputes, and strengthening your bond with your kid all depend on effective communication.

Making Informed and Intentional Parenting Choices: Reflective parenting equips you to make deliberate choices that support your objectives, beliefs, and aspirations as a parent. It supports you as you negotiate challenging parenting situations, make tough decisions, and modify your strategy to fit your child's changing requirements.

Techniques for Examining Your Development as a Parent

Journaling: Write down your emotions, ideas, and observations about your experiences as a parent in a journal or diary. Write about the experiences, obstacles, and realizations you've had along the journey. Examine your diary entries regularly to monitor your development and spot any themes or trends.

Mindfulness Practices: To develop present-moment awareness and nonjudgmental acceptance of your thoughts and emotions as a parent, practice mindfulness exercises like meditation, deep breathing, or mindful awareness. Being mindful helps you become more self-aware and emotionally regulated by enabling you to watch your thoughts and feelings without responding on impulse.

Get Input: Consult dependable friends, relatives, or mentors in parenting for their constructive opinions and insights on your style of parenting. Accept criticism with humility and thankfulness, seeing it as a chance for development and education.

Professional Support: If you're having trouble reflecting on your experiences as a parent, think about getting advice from a therapist, counselor, or parenting coach. They may provide a safe and accepting environment. Expert assistance may provide insightful advice, practical tips, and helpful tools to promote your development and well-being.

Advantages of Examining Your Development as a Parent

Enhanced Self-Awareness and Self-Understanding: Reflective parenting helps you become more aware of your strengths, weaknesses, and opportunities for personal development as a parent.

Better Parenting Skills: You may find areas for growth and hone your parenting abilities to better fulfill your child's requirements by taking a close look at your parenting choices and practices. It also gives you the ability to face obstacles and disappointments with more poise, patience, and understanding.

Stronger Parent-child Connection: By practicing mindfulness and introspection as a parent, you build a closer connection and understanding with your kid that promotes respect, trust, and empathy.

Positive Role Modeling: By setting an example of thoughtful conduct and self-awareness, you help your kid understand the value of self-reflection, personal development, and progress throughout life. This will help them on their path of self-discovery and personal improvement.

As we consider the teachings and perspectives presented in this book, let us keep in mind that being an excellent parent doesn't mean being flawless; rather, it means being there for our kids with love, compassion, and an openness to change and develop. It's about fostering their special abilities and qualities, being aware of and receptive to their needs, and providing them with patience, and understanding guidance as they go through childhood and adolescence.

Asking yourself thoughtful questions might help you go further into self-reflection and self-discovery. For instance:

What parenting skills do I have, and how can I use them to help my child?

What are some of the difficulties I've faced as a parent, and what have I learned from them?

What parenting styles do I want to adopt in light of my realizations and insights?

What long-term objectives do I have for my kid and myself, and how might I go about accomplishing them?

Let's end this chapter and begin the journey of parenting with bravery, and steadfast faith in our capacity to be the greatest parents we can be. May we constantly aim for parenting perfection, knowing that our children deserve nothing less, and may we approach each day with open hearts, ready to welcome the pleasures and difficulties that lie ahead.